ROUTLEDGE LIBRARY EDITIONS:
AGING

Volume 5

DRUGS,
AGEING AND SOCIETY

DRUGS, AGEING AND SOCIETY

Social and Pharmacological Perspectives

BRUCE BURNS
AND
CHRIS PHILLIPSON

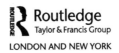

Routledge
Taylor & Francis Group

LONDON AND NEW YORK

First published in 1986 by Croom Helm Ltd

This edition first published in 2024
by Routledge
4 Park Square, Milton Park, Abingdon, Oxon OX14 4RN

and by Routledge
605 Third Avenue, New York, NY 10158

Routledge is an imprint of the Taylor & Francis Group, an informa business

British Library Cataloguing in Publication Data
A catalogue record for this book is available from the British Library

ISBN: 978-1-032-67433-9 (Set)
ISBN: 978-1-032-68777-3 (Volume 5) (hbk)
ISBN: 978-1-032-68781-0 (Volume 5) (pbk)
ISBN: 978-1-032-68780-3 (Volume 5) (ebk)

DOI: 10.4324/9781032687803

Publisher's Note
The publisher has gone to great lengths to ensure the quality of this reprint but points out that some imperfections in the original copies may be apparent.

Disclaimer
The publisher has made every effort to trace copyright holders and would welcome correspondence from those they have been unable to trace.

DRUGS, AGEING and SOCIETY

SOCIAL & PHARMACOLOGICAL PERSPECTIVES

BRUCE BURNS and CHRIS PHILLIPSON

CROOM HELM
London & Sydney

©1986 Bruce Burns and Chris Phillipson
Croom Helm Ltd, Provident House, Burrell Row,
Beckenham, Kent, BR3 1AT
Croom Helm Australia Pty Ltd, Suite 4, 6th Floor,
64-76 Kippax Street, Surry Hills, NSW 2010, Australia

British Library Cataloguing in Publication Data
Burns, Bruce
    Drugs, ageing and society: social and
    pharmacological perspectives.
    1. Geriatric pharmacology
    I. Title II. Phillipson, Chris
    615.5'8'0880565   RC953.7
    ISBN 0-7099-2096-2

Distributed exclusively in the USA by Sheridan House Inc.,
145 Palisade Street, Dobbs Ferry, NY 10522

Printed and bound in Great Britain
by Billing & Sons Limited, Worcester.

CONTENTS

Preface

To Lynn and Jane

Preface

During the past twenty years prescription and over-the-counter drugs have come to play a major role in the health care of older people. This book reviews the historical background to this development and explores its social and pharmacological implications. The main aim of our study is to provide a critical perspective on drug use together with a framework for developing effective prescribing policies. We do not, in developing our arguments, reject the enormous value of drugs in the treatment of many illnesses affecting older people; we do, however, criticise excessive as well as inappropriate prescribing. Our intention is to provide some practical illustrations of how the harmful effects of drug use can be curtailed.

This book is aimed, in particular, at workers in the health services, for example: doctors, health visitors, district nurses, pharmacists, the professions allied to medicine. However, we also hope that it will be of interest to other groups such as social workers, carers, support groups and older people themselves.

The study falls into three main parts. In part one we review the impact of drugs on older people and consider the role of the medical profession and the drugs industry in responding to the health needs of an ageing population. In part two we explore the use and impact of different types of drugs on older people. Finally, in part three, we discuss prescribing policies and complementary approaches to drugs, particularly within the sphere of health education.

Many people have provided help and support in the preparation of this book. Helen Evers gave some valuable references relating to the history of geriatric medicine. Professor Brian Leonard and Dr. Peter Meyer provided criticisms and comments on early drafts of the text. Ms. Candy Norris supplied invaluable advice and material on aspects of prescribing practice. Library staff at the Royal College of General Practitioners, the Barnes Library, University of Birmingham, and the library at the University of Keele, were immensely helpful with bibliographic queries. Finally, we would pay tribute to the great skill and patience of our typist, Sue Allingham; her resourcefulness and hard work have contributed greatly towards the completion of this text.

PART I: Social and Pharmacological Issues

Chapter 1

PRESCRIBING PRACTICES AND OLDER PEOPLE

Introduction

This chapter will introduce some of the problems faced by
older people in taking modern drugs. We shall examine
patterns of prescribing, the use of drugs in residential
settings, self-medication, and illnesses caused by adverse
reactions to drugs. Most of our attention will be focused on
the various difficulties faced by older people when they are
prescribed drugs. At the same time, we cannot ignore the
many gains which drug therapy has brought in alleviating
suffering in old age. Clearly, many drugs are capable of
improving the quality of life experienced by elderly people,
many of whom face debilitating physical and psychological
illnesses. Unfortunately, even for those drugs that work,
there are invariably costs, side effects or adverse reactions.
This is particularly true with older people. Moreover, we
must also be aware of failures at the level of drug promotion
(see Chapter 3) and medical practice (see Chapter 4); these
failures have themselves contributed to illness and death in
old age.

Prescribing Patterns

In the UK, three-quarters of people aged 75 or over receive
prescribed drugs of some kind. Two-thirds of this age group
receive one to three drugs and one-third four to six drugs
simultaneously (Williamson, 1978). As well as taking more
medication per head, the number of prescriptions for elderly
patients is increasing sharply, over and above the increasing
numbers of older people in the population. In 1982 elderly
people in the UK received 15.9 prescriptions per head
compared with 5.2 for the non-elderly; their prescriptions
were also for longer periods (Committee on Safety of
Medicines, 1985). A 1981 survey of American prescribing
patterns, showed patients aged 65 or over accounted for 31
per cent of all drug mentions (drugs recorded during a

1

patient-physician contact). Patients 65 or over had an average of 11 mentions per person, in comparison with 4.52 for the 40-59 age group, and 2.78 for those 20-39 (Baum et al., 1984).

Repeat prescriptions are particularly common amongst older age groups (Bliss, 1981). Such prescriptions are often made out by ancillary staff, particularly if they are given over a long period (Parish, 1971). Prescriptions written by ancillary staff are associated with a rise in errors of prescribing, a fall in early recognition of adverse drug reactions and of clinical change, and a rise in drug interactions (Sharpe and Kay, 1977).

Law and Chalmers (1976) reviewed the drug prescriptions of 151 patients over the age of 75 years living at home. 87 per cent were on regular drug treatment, with 34 per cent taking three to four drugs each per day. They were prescribed three times the number of drugs that were prescribed for the general population, and there were twice as many women as men on regular drug treatment. In a study of patients 70 years and over in a Birmingham practice, half were on long-term drug therapy, mainly for heart disease, depression and anxiety. A survey by Skoll et al. (1979), on prescribing patterns in a Canadian province, found that drugs acting on the cardiovascular system and drugs acting on the central nervous system accounted for two-thirds of all drugs prescribed for older people.

Braverman, at a conference on prescribing for arthritis in the elderly, reported on an analysis of 2000 admissions of the elderly to hospital: 27 per cent were taking analgesics, 12.4 per cent of the admissions were in part due to their drug treatment - largely diuretics and psychotropics - and in 7.7 per cent the drugs were the sole reason for admission (Pulse, November 28 1981, p.68).

The Institute for Social Studies in Medical Care has carried out a number of surveys on the characteristics of drug prescribing. These indicate that men and women aged 55 and over are more likely than younger people to be taking psychotropic and cardiovascular drugs (Anderson, 1980a,b). In addition the 1977 survey reported some interesting class as well as age differences. For example, working class people aged 55 plus were more likely to be taking drugs for rheumatism than middle class people of similar ages (13 per cent compared with 4 per cent); this probably reflects higher rates of chronic illness amongst working class people (see, for example, Townsend and Davidson, 1982). Anderson, (1980a,b) confirmed the high prevalence of combination drug treatment in the elderly with chronic illness conditions, in particular the combination of psychotropic drugs (those acting primarily on the brain) and diuretics (drugs to promote water loss) and medicines for rheumatism.

Jones and her colleagues reviewed patterns of

prescribing by GPs in Bristol and Cardiff. Their data again showed a consistent age trend: 'that is, older patients who consult are rather more likely to get a prescription form than are younger patients' (Jones et al., 1980, p.120). Particularly striking was the authors' finding that, for women in Cardiff, 31 per cent of those over 65 had received three or more prescriptions over a three month period; this compared with just 12 per cent of women under 45.

Drug Use in Residential and Institutional Settings

The problem of over-prescribing has been found to be particularly acute in residential settings. In a study in the USA, Ingman et al. (1975) showed that psychotropic drugs and analgesics were prescribed primarily for symptoms such as agitation, sleeplessness and pain rather than in relation to a diagnosed condition. The least impaired and most active residents of institutions received most of these drugs. Another study in the USA carried out by the Department of Education, Health and Welfare on nursing home residents in ten states found an average of six prescriptions per patient. Multiple prescribing often involved dangerous combinations. The most frequently prescribed drugs were laxatives (60 per cent), analgesics (51 per cent) and tranquillisers (47 per cent).

Christopher et al. (1978) reviewed drug use on geriatric wards in Dundee Hospitals. They found an average of four drugs per patient. These included hypnotics for more than 70 per cent, laxatives for 42 per cent and diuretics for 35 per cent. They found little evidence that the hypnotic drug dosage was reduced with increasing age, thus allowing for the greater sensitivity to these drugs in old age.

Morgan and Gilleard (1981), in their survey of patterns of hypnotic prescribing and usage in 23 residential homes for the elderly in Scotland, found one-third of residents had been given hypnotics (mainly nitrazepam) on the night of the survey, and that half of these were already taking other centrally acting drugs (psychotropics).

Wade et al. (1983) reported the findings of a DHSS funded survey. She examined 794 elderly people selected at random from a number of different care settings. These included 16 local authority homes, 7 voluntary and 7 private residential homes and 8 private nursing homes. Patients in the community were also included, selected at random from the lists of patients of 12 consultant physicians in geriatric medicine who were being attended by community nurses.

The number of drugs taken in the preceding 24 hours was recorded in the survey. Patients in the care of community nurses were the lowest consumers. At the other extreme, of patients in private nursing homes (who were of similar dependency to those in hospital geriatric wards), almost half received four or more drugs, with an average of 3.4 drugs per patient. Differences in types of drug also existed. For example, 27 per cent of hospital patients received laxatives, a figure which was much higher than that found in other settings. However, the most striking differences existed in the use of psychotropic drugs in the 24 hours before the survey. One quarter of patients in private nursing homes received two or more different psychotropic drugs. Women received more than men, but there was no consistent pattern with regard to their level of dependency. There seems to be no satisfactory explanation for the vast diversity in the use of psychotropic drugs: from 18 per cent in the elderly at home supervised by a community nurse to the 78 per cent amongst those in private nursing homes.

The prolific use of psychotropic drugs has serious implications. It has been suggested that the most common iatrogenic illness amongst older people necessitating hospital admission is the result of the cumulative toxic effects of major tranquillising drugs (Bliss, 1981). These effects include various forms of parkinsonism, postural hypotension (sudden falls of blood pressure), drowsiness, confusion, skin rashes and jaundice.

Over-the-Counter Medicines

There is increasing awareness of the large scale nature of over-the-counter (OTC) drug use amongst the elderly and the inevitable increase in drug interactions (Kofoed, 1986). In Dunnell and Cartwright's (1972) UK survey 2 out of 3 old people were found to have taken an OTC drug in the fortnight immediately prior to being questioned. A study by Adams and Smith (1978) showed that 40 per cent of older people in their study practised self-medication during a 48 hour period, and about 80 per cent over a one year period. Much of this self-medication will be unknown to the GP (Taylor, 1983). The practice of self-medication appears to increase with advanced age and be more common amongst women.

Many of the drugs sold to old people over the counter are analgesics. Age in itself modifies the body's handling of these drugs. In addition, smoking appears to antagonise the action of analgesics and to lower the pain threshold in older patients. Pain and hypochondriasis are also common modes of presentation of depressive illness in the elderly which may precipitate a rush to self-medication with analgesics. Drugs to regulate bowel habit are taken in large quantities by older people. Sometimes the altered habit may itself be due to a prescribed drug. Excessive passage of stools can lead to an abnormal loss of potassium and thence induce delirium, whereas impacted faeces can likewise produce a confusional state from dehydration.

Many other examples exist of adverse reactions and interactions from over-the-counter medicines. A large number of remedies for coughs and colds (including nasal sprays) normally contain a combination of cough suppressant (e.g. codeine), antihistamine and a sympathomimetic decongestant. Although often believed to be harmless their use is not without risk mainly caused by the sympathomimetic ingredients. These include ephedrine or ephedrine-like substances which stimulate alpha and beta adrenoreceptors, and which if taken in high doses can increase blood pressure, heart rate and sweating.

Finally, it might also be noted that many of the symptoms from OTC drugs may go unrecognised or may be misinterpreted by the doctor. Moreover, patients who are on several other drugs from their doctor may suffer drug interactions, again without the doctor's awareness.

Drug Induced Disease in the Elderly

A simple definition of an adverse drug reaction is 'any unintended or undesired consequence of drug therapy' (Martys, 1979). Any drug may produce unwanted, unexpected adverse or unpleasant reactions. In other words, there are risks in all forms of drug therapy. It can be said that every individual's drug treatment is an experiment which needs close monitoring. This view is particularly important for those patients who are either very young or very old. Patients aged 60-70 have, in fact, double the rate of adverse reactions compared with those aged under 50. Only a minority of older patients are likely to be warned about the dangers of the drugs they are taking. Thus, a national pharmacy survey found that side effects were mentioned in only 25 per cent of prescriptions given to older people. In addition, 42.5 per cent of the older people surveyed reported that they would not know how to cope with adverse reactions if they occurred (Bosson and Dunn, 1986).

Caird (1977a) argues that the most important single cause of iatrogenic (doctor-induced) disorders in old age is the improper prescription and ingestion of drugs; and in similar vein Bliss (1981) sees older people today as the main 'victims' of modern drugs. He includes as the reasons for this, first, that many doctors lack training in prescribing for older people, and, secondly, the dual prescribing systems in hospitals and in general practice, which prevent doctors from being fully responsible for their own prescribing.

Hurwitz (1969a), in assessing predisposing factors in adverse reactions to drugs, found significantly more patients of 60 years and over and more women than men developing such reactions. Patients who developed adverse reactions were found to have been given more drugs than those who did not. Also significant was a previous history of adverse

5

reactions. In a further analysis of admission to two hospitals in Belfast due to adverse reactions, Hurwitz (1969b) found that they were significantly older than other admissions.

Spiers et al. (1984) analysed the reports of adverse reactions sent to the Committee on Safety of Medicines (CSM), the yellow card system, in the years 1973-1982. When broken down into 5 year periods, 1973-77 and 1978-82, they found that reporting for extremes of age (those under one year and those over 75 years) had increased more rapidly than for children, young and middle-aged adults. In about half the reports the patient was taking one drug only; the rest were taking 2 or more. Fourteen per cent mention 5 or more concurrent drugs. Non-steroidal anti-inflammatory drugs (NSAIDs), used mainly for arthritis, were the most frequently reported class of drug contributing to about one quarter of the total input of reports. Spiers et al. commented that so many reports in one class of drugs should allow for an assessment of comparative safety between drugs in this class. They also found a high rate of reports of adverse reaction with anti-hypertensive drugs, tranquillisers, hypnotics and antidepressants.

In an intensive hospital monitoring report, Hurwitz and Wade (1969) found drug reactions in 10.2 per cent of 1160 patients who received drug treatment. Most reactions were due to the known pharmacological action of the drugs. Only four were life threatening, but 80 were of moderate severity. Digitalis preparations had the highest reaction rate (20 per cent), especially where they were combined with diuretics when the figure reached 24 per cent. With digitalis preparations they found that the rate was highest both totally and relatively in the 60-80 year age band. From their findings they indicated concern about the excessive rates of adverse drug reactions especially amongst older people, but they did point out that if modern potent drugs are to be used in medicine it is inevitable that some adverse reactions will occur.

Martys (1979) studied 817 patients (of all age groups) over a two year period. He found that as many as 41 per cent were thought to have 'certainly' or 'probably' had a reaction to the drug prescribed. Drugs acting on the central nervous system (psychotropic drugs) were responsible for a greater incidence of more severe reactions than drugs in any other group. This has obvious implications for older people, given the frequency with which they are prescribed these drugs (see Chapter 5).

Martys acknowledges that his study among 19 Oxfordshire GPs was a short term survey and that it did not attempt to measure the incidence of side effects in patients on long-term treatment. He felt that he had only skimmed the problem and that additional information was needed on the burden of drug-induced disease in the community.

The voluntary reporting of adverse reactions is a major problem. Melville and Johnson (1982) summarise some of the deficiences associated with the voluntary process of recording adverse reactions (the yellow card system). Spiers et al. (1984), when collating all reports from the years 1972-80, expressed real concern at the absence of any reports from 80 per cent of those doctors eligible to report. There is as yet no large-scale in-depth survey of drug-induced disease in the community, nor does the possibility for daily review exist as in the case of hospital in-patients.

Few studies exist on deaths caused by drugs, but one such study was done in Sweden when 274 drug-induced deaths over a 10 year period were analysed (Bottiger et al., 1979). The researchers found a very marked increase with age in the incidence of fatal reactions. There were more women (60 per cent) than men among drug-induced deaths. However, this over-representation is the same for all adverse drug reactions and corresponds with a proportionately larger drug consumption amongst older women. Increasing age was also found to predispose to more severe drug reactions. It seems of special importance to keep the number of drugs given simultaneously as low as possible - particularly amongst older people. Large numbers of the patients included in the report by Bottiger et al. had been taking many drugs other than the one believed to be responsible for death. Twenty per cent of the patients had been taking 4 drugs or more; the highest figure was 14 drugs taken simultaneously.

Williamson and Chopin (1980) report than an estimated 4000 admissions per year to geriatric units in the UK are due to adverse drug reactions and that these reactions continue to be a major cause of morbidity in the elderly. Behind these statistics lie a number of problems in current general practice. Jarvis (1981), for example, notes the failure to make complete assessments of symptoms, such as insomnia which might be due to a whole range of conditions, from the mundane (a worn-out mattress) to conditions such as depression and incontinence. The use of hypnotics may lead to even more incontinence, restless nights and sometimes to confusional states.

Swollen ankles may also be incompletely assessed. These are often falsely attributed to heart failure when they are more frequently due to immobility, varicose veins, hypoproteinaema (low protein levels in the blood) or impacted faeces. In such instances, diuretics are ineffective and may even make things worse, in that the patient may become dehydrated, confused and incontinent.

Drug treatment is frequently continued for longer than is necessary. Hospital doctors in training grades are reluctant to stop or reduce medication at follow-up clinics. Likewise, general practitioners, given insufficient information from hospital consultants as to when and how medication should be reduced or terminated, continue to prescribe. If the medication is for an indefinite period, this should be clearly stated and the options discussed with the patient, including the targets of minimum dosage which might be achieved with time.

Many diseases are episodic, such as cardiac failure, (provoked for example by a chest infection) and therefore do not need long-term treatment. Among older people, confusional states and depression may arise as a result of physical treatments or changed social circumstances, hence treatment should be continued only as long as the cause persists. Many diseases run an intermittent course with relapses and remissions, e.g. rheumatoid arthritis, bronchitis, depression, various skin disorders. In general, drugs should be continued only as long as necessary, any longer and adverse effects will follow inevitably, some may even mimic the original disease. Sometimes the problem is exacerbated where elderly people mistakenly cling to their tablet routine for security and as a demonstration of their own efforts to combat illness.

Conclusion

All drugs tend to be more dangerous in older people because of misunderstandings of medical treatment schedules, an increase in inter-current illness and impaired liver and kidney function. The elderly are two to three times more likely to suffer harm from medicines than younger people (George, 1981), and the mortality from this form of iatrogenic disease rises exponentially with age. There are many factors that contribute to this high incidence of adverse reactions to drugs. Amongst these we would include inadequate diagnosis, uncritical assessment of the need for treatment, excessive prescribing combined with a tendency for repeat prescriptions to replace clinical reasessment, altered drug handling and increased sensitivity to many drugs in old age. Problems for older people are further exacerbated by the biological changes which accompany the ageing process. It is to a consideration of these that we now turn.

Chapter 2

PHARMACOLOGICAL ISSUES AND OLDER PEOPLE

Introduction

The use of drugs with older people is complicated by a number of factors. First, body tissues in older people undergo changes which mean that they handle and respond to drugs differently in comparison to younger people. Secondly, several major or minor physical diseases may be present at the same time. Thirdly, poor nutrition (a significant problem amongst some groups of older people) may contribute to adverse drug reactions. These problems have to be taken into account when prescribing, in order to reduce the high rate of undesired side effects. Undesirable effects are particularly common with certain groups of drugs. Amongst these we can include psychotropic drugs (minor and major tranquillisers and other drugs that have their primary site of action in the central nervous system); drugs acting on the cardio-vascular system, in particular those for high blood pressure; and analgesics, especially the non-steroidal anti-inflammatory drugs (NSAIDs) used for arthritis.

More research is required regarding altered drug handling (pharmacokinetics) in older people. Speaking very generally, though, a smaller dose of a drug will produce the same effect as the higher 'normal' dose for a younger person. Unfortunately, the situation is not straightforward. For example, it seems that different drugs - even those within the same general group - are handled differently as a factor of age.

Most detailed drug studies are made after single doses in young and usually healthy volunteers. This means that there are very few long-term large-scale studies amongst older people, particularly the frail elderly. There remains a shortage of basic information for the clinician on how their patients will handle many commonly used drugs (such as digoxin) should the patient be old, sick and poorly nourished. Therefore every time a different drug is prescribed for such patients it has to be seen, as was suggested in Chapter 1, as a unique experiment and monitored with the utmost clinical judgement.

Organ function slowly becomes impaired with age. However, this can be very variable, since the ageing process affects people in different ways. In general there is a decline, among people in their 60s and above, in the reserve capacity of organs such as the heart, liver and kidneys. For example, kidney function is reduced by about a half between 20 and 90 years of age;[1] this decline in function being particularly rapid in very elderly people. Initially, the majority of drugs are broken down in the liver by enzymes to inactive substances. These substances in turn, and sometimes the active drug itself, are expelled from the body via the kidneys. Because of a decline in the capacity of the kidneys, there may be a narrowing of the safety margin between the therapeutic and toxic dose of many drugs. Therefore older people, despite wide variations, have a greater tendency to toxic reactions, overdosing and drug interactions. A 'normal' dose for the young could in an old person result in accumulation of the drug if given over a longer period; this may transform a well individual into one who is confused and perhaps incontinent.

Drug Handling in Old Age

In order to gain more understanding of the increased vulnerability of the elderly to drugs, it is necessary to consider some basic pharmacological principles. The effect of any drug upon a cell or tissue is a function of its concentration in its active form at the site of action, together with the sensitivity of the tissue to that drug. The study of what determines this concentration, how long certain concentrations last, and the general passage of a drug through the body, is known as pharmacokinetics. Pharmacokinetics is basically a mathematical analysis of the way the body handles pharmacological agents. It involves the study of drug absorption, distribution, and breakdown into inactive and/or active substances and the subsequent excretion from the body.

Drug Absorption

Most drugs are taken orally and no consistent change in the rate or amount of drug absorbed from the gastrointestinal tract has been shown with ageing. However, reduced absorption of iron (leading to anaemia), calcium and certain vitamins has been demonstrated. Older patients are quite likely to receive more than one drug at a time and the effect of one may substantially affect the absorption of another (e.g. iron and antibiotics). Delayed stomach emptying and hence absorption can occur from drugs that affect the movement of the gut, for example antiparkinsonian and antidepressant drugs. Delayed emptying may in turn increase the irritating affect on the stomach of another drug which has been taken concurrently.

Drug Distribution

After absorption drugs first pass through the liver and are then distributed to other parts of the body. One factor causing an excessive response to standard drug doses is the tendency of the body, in old age, to shrink in size. Older people, in fact, tend to have a smaller body mass, a decline in muscle bulk, a fall in body water, and a disproportionate increase in body fat. Reduced body weight and reduced body water lead to higher drug concentrations in the blood plasma. This is especially the case with water-soluble drugs, e.g. digoxin and the beta-blocker propranolol (Inderal). On the other hand, the relative increase of body fat in old age may lead to a greater volume of distribution and delay in excretion of fat-soluble drugs such as diazepam (Valium).

In their passage through the body, drugs are usually bound to proteins. Serum albumen is the most important of these but it declines with age - particularly where there is disease or malnutrition. When drugs are attached to serum albumen they are inactive. The active component of the drug is the free non-bound fraction, which is usually very small. This free active component that can pass through cell membranes is thus frequently raised in older people to produce a greater effect on the tissues. A potentially dangerous situation also occurs when several different drugs are given at the same time which all compete for the limited amount of available albumen.

A measure of drug breakdown is the time taken for the drug to reach half its highest level in the plasma. This measure is called the drug half-life and is related to the amount of drug available for elimination and to the clearance of the drug by all routes. The half-life is a useful indication of the duration of the effect expected of the drug. With the tissue changes (consequent on ageing) that we have already mentioned there is an increased volume of distribution of drugs, that is a wider spread throughout the body. This results in an extended half-life, or delay in elimination of the drug and the increased hazard of drug accumulation, accentuating and prolonging the response to the drug. For example, because of a greater proportion of fat in the elderly body, fat-soluble drugs like diazepam (Valium) become more widely distributed. As a result, its rate of elimination declines steadily, so that its plasma half-life in hours is prolonged and approximates in hours to the patient's age in years (Klotz et al., 1975). Diazepam is further converted into an active metabolite, desmethyldiazepam, which has an extremely long half-life (that is longer than diazepam). This metabolite can itself accumulate and have an excessively long duration of action in the old and very old.

Drug Breakdown

In the case of older people, considerable reserve capacity in the organs of the body can be lost without significant clinical symptoms. Most drugs are broken down or metabolised in the liver; however, this organ decreases in mass by about 30 per cent between young adulthood and old age. With a decline in cardiac output, blood flow through the liver also declines with age. Metabolism or drug breakdown to inactive substances in the liver is a two-stage process and may be delayed in older people who have a particular illness. Initially, under the influence of certain enzymes, several chemical processes occur to start inactivating the drug. In the second stage the resulting product is combined with substances already in the liver to a water-soluble form and then excreted.

Much of this breakdown occurs during the drug's first passage through the liver after absorption from the gut. All drugs are transported to the liver from the gut via the portal circulation. In old age those drugs that are usually rapidly broken down by the liver may pass unscathed, leading to higher levels reaching the general circulation.

Plasma levels of many drugs after oral administration have been found to be higher in older in comparison with younger patients (e.g. paracetamol, sulphamethiazole, amylobarbitone and propranolol). Propranolol, a potent beta-blocker drug that slows the heart, would normally undergo considerable breakdown on its first passage through the liver. In the elderly, however, there is a reduced breakdown and consequently a potentially toxic level of biologically available drug may reach the heart and elsewhere in the general circulation (Castleden et al., 1975). Slower metabolism in the liver will therefore lead to higher plasma and tissue levels and longer half-lives with the inevitable chance of increased toxic effects (O'Malley et al., 1971).

Some of the wide differences in the effect of drugs in the elderly patient relate to differences of diet. Poor diet and nutrition may increase the risk of toxicity to drugs (Prescott, 1979). Sub-clinical dietary deficiencies in many older patients have been documented; these can in turn be exacerbated by chronic drug administration (Lamy, 1980a). Deficiencies of protein, vitamins, minerals and polyunsaturated fats can all influence enzyme activity in the liver and hence the speed of breakdown of drugs. The influence of the nutritional state on pharmacokinetics in older people has not been fully explored and needs further study (Royal College of Physicians, 1984).

Excretion

There is overwhelming evidence, particularly amongst the very old, of a significant decline in kidney function. The practical importance of this decline for the prescribing of drugs cannot be over-emphasised. Kidney function decreases steadily with age (from maturity onwards). The rate of excretion of drugs tends to decrease in parallel. Changes in drug elimination rates are most important for those drugs where the difference between the therapeutic and the toxic dose is small, e.g. digoxin, hypoglycaemic agents and some antibiotics. Many of the conditions more prevalent in older people, such as heart failure and parkinsonism, need treatment with drugs that have a narrow margin between therapeutic and toxic doses. Defective elimination means that the tissue concentration and therefore the pharmacological effect of most drugs is greater for a given dose. This is one of the main causes for the increased level of adverse reactions to drugs. The risk of these adverse reactions should loom large in any thoughtful consideration of prescribing for this age group, yet many doctors, including general practitioners, may not be fully aware of this (Knox, 1980).

Kidney disease (even a urinary tract infection) and consistent falls of blood pressure, including those from hypotensive drugs or heart failure, can radically reduce kidney function still further and hence the excretion of drugs. A common standard and easy measure of kidney function is the serum creatinine level. Unfortunately, serum creatinine levels may not be an accurate reflection of renal function in the elderly as creatinine production (a function of total muscle mass) falls with age. Creatinine levels, therefore, tend to be low in the elderly with normal or slightly impaired renal function, but if corrected for body weight correlate quite well with the excretory power of the kidneys.

Drug Response in Old Age

Pharmacodynamics refers to the response or effect of a given concentration of a drug at its site of action. These sites may vary in sensitivity to a given drug concentration, and they may also vary with increased age.

Evidence for an altered sensitivity to drugs in older people is limited, primarily because of the absence of research in this field. One example is the effect of sedative and hypnotic drugs on the elderly brain.[2] A greater and more prolonged effect has been found, after psychometric testing, following the ingestion of a single dose of nitrazepam (Mogadon), despite the absence of differences of absorption or excretion of the drug shown by serum levels (Castleden et al., 1977). This is consistent with the clinical observation that a standard dosage for younger patients (5-10 mg) of nitrazepam can produce prolonged confusion by day in some elderly patients (Evans and Jarvis, 1972). Compared with the younger person with the same blood level of, say, diazepam there is a far greater depression of the central nervous system, a greater fall in psychomotor performance and an increase in drowsiness, morning hangover and risk of confusion. Where more than one psychotropic drug is used at the same time the situation is compounded.

Confusional states are increasingly more drug-induced than presenting as part of a disease process (Crammer et al., 1982). Increased sensitivity of the brain, particularly in the very elderly, to standardised blood levels is not restricted to sedatives, but includes such other drugs as the major tranquillisers or neuroleptics, anti-parkinsonian drugs and digoxin. One common end result is a state of confusion or clouded conciousness. Besides confusional states, apparent dementia, depression, incontinence and falls may result.

These unwanted effects may develop insidiously over months, or even after years on long-term therapy, because of increased brain sensitivity or very slow accumulation of a drug or both. Recognition may then be difficult because deterioration develops insidiously and there may be no obvious improvement for several days after the drug is stopped. The patient and the doctor may often be unaware of these factors.

Other Drug Hazards in Old Age

An additional problem faced by older people is impairment of the mechanisms which control body temperature, heart rate, blood pressure and muscular co-ordination. This fragility of the body's controlling and correcting mechanisms can be made worse by certain drugs, especially when taken in combination.

Old people cope less well with extremes of cold or heat. Drugs such as the major tranquillisers blunt their ability to regulate body temperature. Whereas in the younger patient temperature regulation is maintained, in the older person significant clinical change such as severe hypothermia may result. This can occur even when it is not particularly cold, especially if the patient remains very still. Of course immobility and reduced levels of consciousness are readily achieved in old people by tranquillisers, independent of the blunting effect that the drug has on the central temperature-regulating mechanism.

Another susceptibility met frequently among older people is that to sudden or prolonged falls in blood pressure (postural hypotension); these are all too frequently induced by many of the widely differing groups of drugs commonly used today. Typically these catastrophic falls of pressure, which fail to be corrected, occur when the patient stands up quickly. The baroreceptors, or pressure receptors, in the artery walls (which control blood pressure) are simply less efficient. Drugs such as major tranquillisers, antidepressants, diuretics and beta blockers are some of many that can easily induce postural hypotension, with consequent dizziness, fainting and falls.

Multiple pathology is the rule in geriatric medicine. The clean-cut, single diagnosis that the young doctor is trained to make becomes an altogether more blurred operation in older age groups. Physical disorders are also likely to be common. A list might include heart failure, organic brain disease, Parkinson's disease, renal failure, liver failure, arthritis, prostate enlargement, constipation, diabetes, infections and hypertension. Multiple symptoms and signs invite multiple drug treatments. Polypharmacy becomes the order of the day, yet the incidence of adverse drug reactions increases dramatically with the number of drugs taken.

With multiple drug prescribing goes a high prevalence of errors in compliance. The situation is often compounded by self-medication, sensory loss, loss of mobility of the joints, and mental confusion. Caird has argued, with regard to multiple drug prescribing, that

> the number of drugs that individual old people are expected to take is inversely proportional to the amount of thought given to the problem by their doctors. Even though the multiple pathology of the elderly constitutes a standing temptation to polypharmacy, many of the drug regimes on which old people are both discharged from and admitted to hospital provide better evidence of prescribers' enthusiasm than of their common sense (Caird, 1977a, p.612).

Conclusion

Older people may differ from younger people in the quantity of the drug presented at the target organ (pharmacokinetics), the sensitivity of the organ to the drug (pharmacodynamics) and their principal compensatory mechanisms against the effect of the drug. Associated degenerative diseases are common in the very elderly which in turn affect drug handling and response, as does the practice of giving several drugs at the same time.

If one can generalise, biological changes in organ systems lead to higher concentrations of drugs in the plasma and tissues. In addition, potent concentrations of drugs last for a much longer duration. That is, for many drugs increasing age prolongs their half-lives, a measure of the rate of elimination of the drug and indirectly of how long the drug is likely to have its effect. There is great individual variability (especially among older people), and each patient has to be monitored individually. Older people should be started on smaller doses, preferably single drug regimes, and should be seen regularly, especially in the early days of therapy.

It is important to remember that very few drugs have a specific dosage recommended for older people. Dosage regimes for new drugs including those specifically offered to older people (e.g. anti-arthritic drugs) are still established on data which are largely obtained from younger often fitter people.

Having stated, for much of this chapter, some negative aspects of ageing, it is perhaps salutory to remind ourselves that the broader context of ageing is more positive. Dovenmuehle, writing in the first collection of reports from the Duke University longitudinal study of ageing, summarises the research evidence as follows:

> Although disease disability cannot be completely avoided with the passage of time, especially after the sixtieth year, there is good evidence to indicate that relative preservation of health and of ability to carry out one's life activities can be attained with adequate medical care. Much of this care has to be concentrated upon the physical aspects of illness and disability, but there is also room for considerably more effort toward improving the accompanying depression associated with illness (Dovenmuehle, 1970, p.47).

For the rest of part one of this book, we shall examine the role of drug companies and the medical profession in the development of 'adequate medical care'.

Footnotes

1. For a more detailed discussion of these changes, see the following: Crooks, O'Malley and Stevenson (1976), Vestel (1978) and Rogers, Spector and Trounce (1981).
2. For further reading on this area see Hicks et al., (1982).

Chapter 3

OLDER PEOPLE AND THE DRUGS INDUSTRY

Introduction

Chapters one and two highlighted the vulnerability of older people to side effects and adverse reactions from drugs. Our analysis indicated the need for careful monitoring in the use of drugs, and for caution when new products are prescribed. Yet the reality is that these conditions are often not met and that, in consequence, older people have had often to face considerable problems when using drugs. These problems have been exacerbated by, first, a pharmaceutical industry anxious to increase its profits, secondly, weaknesses in controls from regulatory bodies and, thirdly, negative attitudes within the medical profession. A combination of these factors has helped to create a climate of risk and uncertainty for older people seeking medical care. In this chapter we focus upon the problems created by the rise of the drug industry; in chapter 4 we examine the relationship between older people and the medical establishment.

Older People and the Drugs Market

Older people are, in an important sense, both products and victims of the rise of the modern drugs industry. The application of modern pharmacology has undoubtedly stimulated improvements in mortality and morbidity. A publication from the Office of Health Economics (a body founded in 1962 by the Association of the British Pharmaceutical Industry) argues that: 'The difference in trends for the years from the 1940s to the 1970s indicates that a quarter of a million people are alive today who would have died during their childhood had there been no improvement in mortality due to modern pharmacology' (Office of Health Economics (OHE), 1980, p.10).

Many pensioners would undoubtedly be dead or, at the very least, extremely ill, were it not for some of the major post-war successes in the drugs field. However, the companies themselves would be substantially poorer without the massive market provided by older people. In many cases it has been the financial attraction of sales in this sector which has been a guiding influence for companies, the prospects of major financial gains blurring an appreciation of the dangers of pharmaceutical drugs to elderly consumers.

The market is an impressive one. In a single month, in Britain, over ten million prescriptions are likely to be made out to people of pensionable age, and older people receive twice as many prescriptions as the national average. But the protection for older people against adverse side-effects is often inadequate. The Royal College of Physicians, in their report Medication for the Elderly, commented that:

> .... clinical pharmacological studies with new drugs are usually conducted on young, healthy subjects and pre-marketing clinical trials rarely involve significant numbers of old and very old patients. Consequently, manufacturers' data sheet information on the safety and efficacy of new drugs in the elderly is often inadequate (Royal College of Physicians, 1984, p.6).

This statement was made 21 years after the formation of the Committee on Safety of Medicines (CSM), formed in the wake of the thalidomide scandal; and 13 years after the introduction of the Medicines Act which requires that all new drugs be scrutinised for safety, quality and efficacy. Unfortunately, these controls, which are weaker in Britain than in many other countries,[1] have proved vulnerable to various kinds of pressure exercised by drug companies. This pressure has become more intense as the companies have faced a squeeze on their profits. This has arisen for a variety of reasons: the cut-backs in government spending, the ending of patents on money-spinning drugs, and the failure to find new super-drugs to boost sales. Reduced profits have led companies to increase the amount they spend on research and development, and to diversify the work they do in this area. According to one report:

> Instead of specialising on certain market sectors, such as antibiotics or painkillers, in the hope of coming up with a blockbuster pill, companies are diversifying their research to take in most therapeutic categories. Usually this means drugs targeted at the growing population of old people and the progressive or 'chronic' diseases (such as arthritis, cancer and heart disease) (The Economist, 12 January, 1985).

It is the way in which many drugs are 'targeted' that chiefly concerns us in this chapter. Through their activities in education and promotion the companies exercise enormous influence. In this chapter we ask: does this influence always work to the benefit of the older consumer? What sort of pressures are faced by doctors in prescribing to older consumers? What are the problems associated with drug advertising?

Educating Doctors

Shulman (1982) notes that the moment someone becomes a medical student, they become the object of lavish attentions from the drug industry. In the 1950s, the drug companies were 'virtually the only source of information about new medicines on which doctors could base their prescribing decisions' (OHE, 1977, p.5). A survey by Wilson et al. in the 1960s concluded that: 'British general practitioners depend to a large extent on the pharmaceutical industry for information about advances in therapeutics which have occurred since their medical training ceased, and they use this information widely when prescribing for their patients' (Wilson et al., 1963, p.603). By the 1970s, doctors were drawing upon a variety of sources for their knowledge, but with drug companies still of major importance (Eaton and Parish, 1976). This reliance has continued through into the 1980s (Medawar, 1984).

The drug industry has also maintained its intensive marketing strategies, spending around £5000 a year per doctor on promoting its products. Such was the concern at the tactics adopted by some companies that a two year investigation by the Royal College of Physicians was mounted in 1984 into the links between the pharmaceutical industry and the medical profession. The enquiry arose from:

> .... allegations that some doctors and people working in medical research are subject to undue pressure because of the volume of publicity, propaganda and inducements to try out or favour any particular product. In 1981, the average cost of promoting a new pharmaceutical product was about £1.1 million with just over half being spent on advertising. Also likely to come under scrutiny is the amount of clinical pharmacology financially supported by the drug industry which is estimated to support approximately one in six people working in clinical pharmacology departments (Guardian, 27 July, 1984).

General practitioner education has been an important area of work for many firms (Melville and Johnson, 1982). Some companies have their own departments of postgraduate medical education. Through these they produce videotapes in which their products feature or they recommend experts to speak on subjects in which they have a commercial interest

(Paton, 1984, p.8). A number of surveys have confirmed the popularity with GPs of commercially sponsored functions (Pickup et al., 1983; During and Gill, 1974). One clinical pharmacologist has argued that:

> Doctors are becoming so accustomed to sponsored postgraduate education that it is difficult to attract them to meetings where they have to pay for their own registration and refreshments. Postgraduate education is thus tending to become the responsibility of the drug industry rather than of postgraduate deans, clinical tutors, and the profession itself. This trend should be a cause of major concern ... because of the potential for distorting postgraduate medical education away from the needs of patients and the health service, towards the requirements of the industry.

The writer went on to suggest that:

> Most doctors believe that they are quite untouched by the seductive ways of the industry's marketing men; that they are uninfluenced by the promotional propaganda they receive; that they can enjoy a company's 'generosity' in the form of gifts and hospitality without prescribing its products. The degree to which the profession, mainly composed of honourable and decent people, can practise such self-deceit is quite extraordinary. No drug company gives away its shareholders' money in an act of disinterested generosity. Just as research grants are given to meet the costs of producing information of direct relevance to the company, so too is the promotional budget used to persuade doctors to prescribe the company's drugs. The harsh truth is that not one of us is impervious to the promotional activities of the industry, and that the industry uses its various sales techniques because they are effective (Rawlins, 1984, pp.276, 277).

Conferences may be supported without specific mention of a firm's range of products (although the publicity value is still very important). At the other extreme, seminars and meetings may be subsidised solely for the purpose of evaluating - or advertising - a new drug. Subsidised journals are also used to publicise favourable research findings.

The drug representative

The education of the doctor is also maintained through the drug reps: there are 3500 covering the country's 29,000 GPs (i.e. one rep for every 8 GPs). Research indicates that GPs are likely to learn about the existence of a new drug from the rep, and a majority value what he or she has to say about it (Eaton and Parish, 1976). Braithwaite notes that the sales rep is told by the company that he or she has a dual responsibility: 'to sell and promote the advantages of the product, but also to educate doctors as to the risks and limitations of this therapy' (1984, p.224). However, the author goes on to argue that reps are rewarded by the volume of their sales, not their ability to improve the knowledge of physicians. Braithwaite concludes that: 'The pressure to achieve sales makes it difficult for the company representative to be objective in presenting the advantages and disadvantages, compared with alternative therapies, of the product he/she is pushing. Indeed, many representatives discard any pretence of a fair presentation of risks and benefits' (Braithwaite, 1984, p.224).

Current sales techniques were highlighted in a series of bulletins for drug reps employed by Geigy Pharmaceuticals, as reported in the Observer newspaper. The documents illustrated how the company instructed reps to avoid discussing awkward topics, e.g. rumours about problems with adverse side effects associated with a particular drug (the example cited was with an anti-arthritis drug). The bulletins also suggested that the company tried to influence medical opinion by trying to organise the publication of letters championing their drugs in leading medical newspapers. The Observer reported that:

> In June, 1984, when a letter appeared in The Lancet from the University of Florida suggesting that Geigy's drug Transiderm Nitro was ineffective, the company told its reps: 'We are asking Ciba-Geigy USA to reply to this letter as it originated from there. Our medical department is organising a reply from an eminent British source. ON NO ACCOUNT INITIATE A DISCUSSION WITH THE DOCTOR.'
> Within three months, two letters had appeared in The Lancet, replying to the article, one from a British cardiologist and one from Ciba-Geigy Ltd., in Switzerland (Observer, 9 June 1985).

Drug Advertising

In many respects the medical environment is one which is heavily biased towards the products and interests of the pharmaceutical industry. This is nowhere more apparent than in the lucrative world of advertising, an area where the needs of the elderly have, unfortunately, often taken second place in the face of sensational claims for breakthrough drugs. Dubious advertising is not a new problem. A 1962 survey of adverts in medical journals considered that, in 22 out of 45 advertisements, unwarranted claims were made and often serious effects or disadvantages were not mentioned or glossed over (cited in the Sainsbury report, 1967). And the Sainsbury Committee, after examining a range of adverts, commented that: 'most seemed to rely on the common promotional devices to a greater or lesser extent and some seemed more concerned with imprinting a brand name on a doctor's mind than with seriously conveying medical information' (Sainsbury Report, 1967, p.67).

Gillie and La Guardia have argued that many infringements of the law pass unnoticed because the Department of Health does not have a comprehensive system for monitoring drug adverts. Between 1979 and 1984 there were only two prosecutions by the Department of Health, these being for minor offences. They conclude that: 'A misleading advert may run for months before being corrected - and by then it has had an impact on doctors. Even when changes are enforced to correct misleading claims, these are generally made without the publicity clarifying what is happening' (Sunday Times, 13 May 1984).

An unpublished survey by a senior Department of Health official found extensive evidence of drug firms breaking their own code of practice. Some made misleading claims about the benefits of their drugs; others failed to warn doctors of serious side effects. The study also found that some of the scientific references quoted to support the claims were irrelevant, misquoted, or unobtainable (Guardian, 13 September 1984). The last finding is not new. Stimson's 1976 study found a considerable proportion of references in drug adverts were unavailable, either because they were unpublished, or because they were not taken by the kind of library which doctors most often used.

The above problems tend to be magnified in conditions most directly experienced by older people (e.g. heart disease and arthritis), where the drugs market is at its most competitive, and where there is pressure to make exaggerated claims for new products. Certainly, the evidence cited so far must cast some doubt on the view of the OHE that: ' ... the information provided by the manufacturers is now closely controlled both in content and volume' (OHE, 1977, p.23). Indeed, doubt on this has been cast by the industry itself. In 1983 the then president of the Association of the British Pharmaceutical Industry (ABPI) was reported in the minutes of an ABPI meeting to have expressed misgivings about the 'styles of promotion ... adopted by certain companies'. He argued: 'It was not acceptable for chief executives to expect results while turning a blind eye to the methods which their marketing departments adopted in achieving them. The industry's image was damaged by promotional excesses' (Guardian, 9 March 1983).

But does it really matter that, according to Heath and

Miller, modern drug advertising resembles 'the pop-up books so enjoyed by pre-school children'? (Heath and Miller, 1983, p.904). Surely, the argument would run, doctors are too sophisticated to be influenced by the images and slogans of the advertising agencies.

Unfortunately, there is some evidence that doctors may either be unwilling to admit the influence of drug adverts or may lack awareness that they do have an influence. These possibilities were suggested in an American study by Avorn et al., (1982), which reviewed scientific versus commercial influences on prescribing habits. This investigation questioned the value of studies which relied upon the self-reports of doctors to determine the influences on prescribing decisions. As an alternative to self-reporting, the study examined views about certain drugs which had attracted conflicting claims from commercial and non-commercial sources. For example, cerebral and peripheral vasodilators are widely promoted (see Chapter 7) for the treatment of senile dementia. However, the clinical and research literature has concluded that such drugs are of dubious value. Indeed, it is suggested that: 'advertisements for these drugs are the major current sources of the misinformation that mental failure in the elderly is the result of inadequate cerebral blood flow - a concept now abandoned by neurologists ... ' (Avorn et al., 1982, p.5).

Most of the doctors interviewed reported that drug adverts had a 'minimal influence on their prescribing habits'. Yet the study also showed, in relation to cerebral vasodilators, that a majority of those questioned believed that 'impaired cerebral blood flow is a major cause of senile dementia'. The researchers concluded that: 'Although the vast majority of practitioners perceived themselves as paying little attention to drug advertisement and [drug representatives] as compared with papers in the scientific literature, the beliefs about the effectiveness of [cerebral vasodilators] revealed quite the opposite pattern of influence on large segments of the sample' (Avorn et al., 1982, p.7).

How can we explain this variance between the beliefs and the prescribing habits of doctors? Four factors may be cited which help to increase the impact of drug advertising. First, there is evidence that specific campaigns for new drugs can have a disproportionate influence on doctors. Secondly, specific diseases (particularly those of a 'low risk' and chronic nature) may be more susceptible to particular forms of promotion. Third, the sheer volume of publicity emerging from the drug industry undoubtedly helps to concentrate the range of treatment strategies selected by doctors. Finally, drug advertising may reinforce pessimistic medical views about older people and thereby influence the promotion of certain drugs.

The first two points may be illustrated with specific

examples. Advertising for the anti-arthritic drug benoxaprofen (brand name Opren) in Britain cost its manufacturer around £1 million (this was spent within a two-year period). But the impact of this can be measured by the fact that the drug was given, in the two years from its launch to eventual withdrawal, to nearly three-quarters of a million patients, most of these being older people. In the case of another arthritic drug (a new formulation of indomethacin - brand name Osmosin), its manufacturers - Merck, Sharp and Dohme - spent £200,000 in just two months on promotional activities (the drug was later withdrawn from the market after being implicated in 23 deaths). Faced with these saturation campaigns (combined with pressure from patients or relatives) doctors may well be responsive to persuasion from the drug companies.

Of equal importance is the lack of balance in medical advertising. Set beside the industry's promotional budget - £180 million in 1983-84 - the amount spent on prevention and health education is derisory (the annual budget of the Health Education Council is around nine million pounds). Presentations regarding the value of exercise or healthy eating can rarely compete with the insistent claims of drug manufacturers. Indeed, it is important to observe that whereas virtually all medical publications carry drug adverts (and are, in some cases, only financially viable because of them), there are few equivalent adverts, in the medical literature at least, stressing, for example, a health education and health promotion view.

Finally, drug firms may also influence the attitudes of doctors in a more global sense, highlighting age as a negative process marked by inevitable deterioration and suffering (Lehr, 1983). The diffusion of negative stereotypes may itself be important in promoting the sale of pharmaceutical products, producing a narrowing in the range of treatment options considered suitable for older people.

The points being made here are not simply of academic interest. In some instances the tensions described may work against the interests of older people, causing as a result much pain and suffering, even death. The 1980s have seen a number of such examples.

Where the Controls Broke Down

To illustrate some of the problems associated with current marketing techniques, we shall first explore the promotion of NSAIDs which came either to be banned or reviewed by the CSM following their use in the UK. The drugs are benoxaprofen (brand name Opren): 83 deaths - mostly elderly people - plus at least 4000 experiencing serious side effects; slow-release indomethacin (brand name Osmosin): 23 deaths and 400 people with serious side effects; indoprofen (brand name Flosint): 7 deaths and 210 with serious side effects; piroxicam (brand name Feldene): 77 reports of deaths in patients taking piroxicam, plus 2000 people experiencing severe side effects. The number of patients taking these drugs varied from 75,000 (in the case of indoprofen) to 750,000 (in the case of benoxaprofen).

There is undoubtedly a vast market for drugs concerned with treating rheumatic pain. Every year 8 million people consult a GP for some rheumatic problem, accounting for 15 per cent of all patients on each practitioner's list and 23 per cent of all consultations. The total number of prescriptions for NSAIDs issued in the UK rose from 7.6 in 1967 to 22 million in 1985. The increase was particularly marked in the case of the elderly, and it is likely that every individual aged over 65 will on average receive at least one prescription for an NSAID in any one year (Walt et al., 1986).

In terms of prescribing such drugs, the GP is faced with a bewildering range of possibilities. According to George Nuki, of Newcastle University:

> The proliferation of new agents largely reflects the fact that none is ideal and that the market for new products is large and lucrative. In the main, the newer agents are "me too" molecular variants of older aspirin-like drugs. None is appreciably more effective than aspirin in controlling symptoms in patients with inflammatory joint disease, although some are better tolerated and more convenient to take (Nuki, 1983, p.39).

This 'lucrative market' has undoubtedly created considerable temptations for drug manufacturers. This was illustrated in a number of controversies surrounding the four drugs listed above. In the case of benoxaprofen, dubious marketing methods and distortion of scientific evidence have been two of the more serious allegations made against its manufacturer. Introduced into Great Britain in 1980 by an American company, Eli Lilly, it met with enthusiastic press reviews, with promises that it would bring a 'new era' to the treatment of arthritis.[2] Advertisements described the drug as a 'brand new' anti-arthritic agent, one which had only mild side effects and which, most important of all, could actually modify the arthritic disease process. This claim could not actually be checked in the early period of benoxaprofen's use, since the reference to which the reader was directed contained the legend 'awaiting publication'. Given the gravity of the claims for benoxaprofen, this delay was unfortunate. Nonetheless, it did appear that this could be the breakthrough to relieve the suffering of thousands of people.

However, critical findings began to emerge fairly soon after the drug's introduction onto the British market. Just 12 months after the exciting announcements in papers such as

The Times and the Guardian, the Drug and Therapeutics Bulletin published the sober assessment that 'Opren appears no better than other drugs in this category nor effective when the others have failed' (Drug and Therapeutics Bulletin, 1980, p.96). Throughout 1981 and 1982, reports began to accumulate in medical journals about the side-effects of benoxaprofen; these included photosensitivity and gastro-intestinal problems. Ironically, in one of the last issues of the British Medical Journal to carry an advert for the drug (one which showed a delighted old lady carrying her shopping with renewed vigour), there were two major articles reporting serious side-effects arising from its use. One of these articles concluded, '[benoxaprofen] is a potent phototoxic drug and ... the manufacturer's recommended dosage of 600 mg daily is associated with an unacceptable incidence of side-effects in the elderly'. This article appeared in May 1982. By June of that year, doctors were asked to reduce the dose given to older people. Two months later the drug was suspended and in September 1982 Eli-Lilly withdrew the drug from the UK market. By this time 65 people had died and over 3000 had experienced serious side effects.[3]

With the drug being launched on a wave of media publicity,[4] it was to remain in the public eye as reports of side-effects appeared in the national papers. Both the Guardian and The Sunday Times ran a number of reports highlighting the experience of patients receiving the drug. They also carried virtually identical stories alleging that Eli-Lilly had delayed reporting the danger of benoxaprofen to the Department of Health or the Committee on Safety of Medicines (CSM). But the most sustained attack both on the behaviour of Eli-Lilly and on the promotional activities of drug firms came with the BBC Panorama programmes entitled 'The Opren Scandal' (10 and 17 January, 1983).

The programmes identified three scandals associated with the drug: (1) that the manufacturer made a number of dubious claims in its promotional activities, in particular, its assertion that benoxaprofen could 'modify the arthritic process' was at best highly misleading, and based upon a false comparison between changes in rats and possible changes in human beings; (2) that the company withheld details of the large number of patients who had side effects (photosensitivity in particular) during trials of the drug in America; (3) that the company had failed to respond to crucial information about the effects of the drug on its biggest consumer, namely, older people. Research had indicated, as early as 1981, that benoxaprofen was eliminated very slowly from the kidneys of elderly patients. Because of the danger of the drug accumulating in the body, the recommended dosage would need to be at least halved, a proposition which the company viewed as commercially non-viable (it was, in fact, 12 months before this vital recommendation was finally made to doctors in Britain).

In many respects, this third point raises one of the most important issues connected with benoxaprofen. As we have seen, its biggest consumer was always likely to be elderly people. It seems reasonable to suppose, therefore, that they would have been over-represented in trials of the drug. Yet we know that out of the 500 patients tested with benoxaprofen before it received its British licence, just 52 were aged over 65 (Sunday Times, 27 February, 1983). This figure is disturbingly small given: (1) that the elderly are vulnerable to adverse drug reactions and (2) that benoxaprofen had produced significant side-effects in the early stages of testing. Moreover, the problems arising from inadequate testing were compounded by the publicity surrounding the launch of the drug. As Paul Turner (Professor of Clinical Pharmacology at St Bartholomew's Hospital in London) was to point out,

> because the launch of benoxaprofen had received a lot of media publicity patients had tended to ask doctors for the drug. Use of the drug then increased very rapidly so that it became virtually impossible to maintain adequate surveillance on all the patients receiving it. It also meant ... that the drug was used on large numbers of patients for whom it was not really intended (our emphasis) (Pharmaceutical Journal, 1982, p. 214).

One allegation against Eli-Lilly was that they deliberately picked British arthritis sufferers as guinea-pigs for the drug. A former senior marketing man for Eli-Lilly claimed that a plan was drawn up at the firm's Indianapolis headquarters for a massive publicity campaign that would get British patients demanding Opren from their doctors. The place and time of the year were chosen so as to mask the most serious side-effects of the drug. This was the 'photo-toxic' reaction which can cause painful weals after only a few minutes exposure to the sun (Mail on Sunday, 13 February 1984).

Marketing techniques used with benoxaprofen also showed the ambivalence towards doctors expressed by some drug companies. Thus the manual used by the company salesforce had the following instructions:

> Sales reps were instructed to keep the Opren story as simple as possible: 'GPs don't understand the highly technical data on the arthritis inflammatory process,' the Company told its salesmen. 'Even though they talk about PSI activity' (that's an aspect of the illness) 'they don't really understand it.' 'Remember,' salesmen were told, 'sell the product benefits not the science' (Panorama, BBC TV, 17 January 1983).

And, according to a report from the Opren Action Committee:

> Sales representatives were instructed to play down the evidence of the adverse effects of benoxaprofen. They were briefed to say that photosensitivity occurred in about 4% and onycholysis in about 1% of cases, and to stress that these unusual side effects were cosmetic in nature (Opren Action Committee, 1985).

Eli Lilly did eventually admit, in August 1985, to deception with their drug, with the company and its former chief medical officer accepting that they had failed to tell the US authorities about deaths among patients using the drug in Britain. According to a report on the trial of Eli-Lilly in America:

> In January 1982, Shedden and two other doctors at Lilly received from Britain a list of numerous adverse reactions, including 26 cases of serious liver disorders (two of which were fatal) and 23 other fatalities.

> On 5 February 1982, an employee of Lilly who had just visited Britain briefed Shedden and several senior Lilly officials in Indianapolis on foreign experience with the drug. The employee presented a report prepared by Lilly in Britain that tabulated 27 kidney/liver reactions, five of which were fatal (New Scientist, 29 August 1985).

It is now known that around 26 Americans (mostly elderly) died of liver and/or kidney failure after Oraflex (the American version of Opren) was placed on the market. More than 200 patients suffered non-fatal liver and kidney failure during that time.

Indoprofen was another NSAID which arrived (at the beginning of 1983) on a surge of publicity, with GPs being told of its merits in the congenial environment of Henry Ford's yacht. Advertising reported a range of findings demonstrating the drug's superiority over other NSAIDs, with the usual claims being made regarding minimal side-effects. The Drug and Therapeutics Bulletin, however, was soon to report that indoprofen resembled most other NSAIDs in respect of efficacy and adverse effects. Indeed, it concluded that: 'It has no special virtues and is more expensive than even the well-established twice daily NSAIDs' (Drug and Therapeutics Bulletin, 1983, p.88). In fact, barely a year after its launch, the drug was banned by the then Health Minister, Kenneth Clarke. The manufacturers had refused a voluntary withdrawal, despite reports that patients were dying at the rate of almost one every two months, on the basis that this would affect sales in other countries.

The case of indomethacin showed how multi-national companies could combine sales staff from different companies within a corporation, as part of a sustained promotion drive.[5] In November and December 1982 Merck Sharp and Dohme spent in excess of £800,000 directly, and over £120,000 through their subsidiary Thomas Morson, in promoting a new formulation of indomethacin (Osmosin). Thomas Morson were, in fact, the manufacturers of an earlier version of indomethacin (Indocid-R). When Osmosin was withdrawn (amidst allegations that it was tested on insufficient numbers of people to identify serious side-effects), Morson switched to spending heavily on advertising for Indocid-R (Guardian, 7 October 1983).

Finally, piroxicam (brand name Feldene) was the subject of investigation by the CSM in 1986, following a number of research reports suggesting gastro-intestinal side effects. First introduced in 1980, the drug entered the market with the usual claims of minimal side effects, particularly in respect of peptic ulceration. Piroxicam quickly established itself as a brand leader, achieving three million prescriptions issued in 1984 (most of these being given to people over 60). Pfizer, the manufacturer, earned £400 million in 1985 in worldwide sales from piroxicam.

The drug's tendency to cause gastro-intestinal bleeding had been known to the CSM since 1982. In October of that year the Committee sent a warning to doctors about side effects and the company made changes to the prescription advice on piroxicam's data sheet. The company was itself aware of a number of research studies circulating in 1982, suggesting particular side effects. These reports included research by Emery and Grahame (1982) from the department of Rheumatology at Guy's Hospital, London; Morgan et al. at Airdale Hospital, Keighley; and a report from the Norwegian Drug Authority.

In the light of these early investigations, and the warning from the CSM, it is somewhat surprising to find in 1983 that Pfizer were advertising piroxicam as a drug which had a: 'low level of side effects [making] [it] very suitable for the elderly patient' (our emphasis) (Pulse, 9 July 1983). Its 'suitability', however, was to be questioned with increasing frequency over the next few years, with studies from Sweden and Britain suggesting a particular problem with peptic ulceration. By December 1985, the CSM had received 77 yellow card reports of deaths in patients taking piroxicam - most of these, of course, being elderly people. In this context, it is significant that the manufacturer's own guidelines varied from country to country: in Ireland, doctors were given specific warnings about the risks of the drug when given to older people; in Britain and the US, no such warnings were issued.[6]

In fact, contrary to the competing claims made for individual NSAIDs, it is still very difficult to determine whether any one drug is more or less likely to cause severe side effects (Committee on Safety of Medicines Update, 1986). The case of piroxicam shows the danger of inflated promises in the early life of a drug. Six years after its launch - amid claims of a very low incidence of ulcers and blood loss - the CSM is now considering telling doctors to avoid giving piroxicam to elderly arthritic patients, unless nothing else will do. The public itself is caught between conflicting recommendations. The American Health Research Group have argued that 'piroxicam should not be used by people over 60'. The manufacturers, on the other hand, assert that the drug poses no greater risk for the elderly than any other NSAID. In the middle, the CSM put the case for caution when using most brands of anti-arthritics:

> The decision about the appropriateness of treatment with a non-steroidal anti-inflammatory drug in an individual patient must continue to depend on the judgement of the prescribing doctor. In making such risk:benefit judgements doctors should take into account new findings, which strengthen the CSM's view that non-steroidal anti-inflammatory drugs should not be given to patients with active peptic ulceration. In patients with a history of peptic ulcer disease and the elderly they should be given only after other forms of treatment have been carefully considered. Moreover, it is prudent in all patients to start treatment at the bottom end of the dose range. It is salutary to remember that many patients with bleeding or perforated peptic ulcers attributable to non-steroidal anti-inflammatory drugs have had no history of dyspepsia or peptic ulceration (CSM Update, 1986, p. 614).

It is clear, however, that the education of the public about piroxicam leaves much to be desired. It is inexplicable, for example, that the drug should have been advertised as especially suitable for older people some 12 months after warning reports had been received about serious side effects. It is of equal concern that Pfizer should have made representations to two medical journals expressing their objections about articles containing criticisms of piroxicam, which had been submitted for publication.[7] There is surely a need for as open a debate as possible about the advantages and disadvantages of particular drugs. In most cases, it would seem that discussion is heavily weighted towards the former, with very few accessible forums giving a balanced view about the value of drug treatment.[8]

All four drugs under discussion were the subject of major

press campaigns, all of which used conventional advertising techniques to press home their advantages over other drugs. Slogans were one kind of device: benoxaprofen promised the doctor 'A new way of life for your arthritic patients'; indoprofen carried the legend 'Towards mobility without pain', and piroxicam promised 'continuous relief with a single daily dose'. The 'tests show' marketing ploy was another popular tactic, with dramatic diagrams and figures illustrating the superiority of a particular drug over other anti-arthritic agents.

Even though the elderly were likely to be major consumers of the drugs, only one (benoxaprofen) featured an older person in its advertising campaign. The drug's depiction of a delighted elderly consumer was somewhat ironic given the alleged suppression by the company that this age group could not tolerate the recommended dosage of the drug.

However, we can detect more general problems with drug advertising. Obviously the information in advertising is abridged data. In theory, it should adhere to the indications in the officially approved data sheet. Few companies are likely to risk presenting discrepant data, though examples can be found where this has been done (as with tiaprofenic acid - see below). The problem with many presentations relates to their focusing on unreliable or unproven data; or failing to give clarity about particular advantages or disadvantages to certain groups.

On the question of the advantages and disadvantages of drugs, present practice leaves much to be desired. Thus, prescribing information on advertisements in the case of NSAIDs typically cautions against use in pregnancy. But why stop here? Given the precautions necessary when using NSAIDs with the elderly, why not list some of the particular problems with this age group? Companies may fail to do this because of insufficient data or because it would mean qualifying marketing claims. Either way, adverts present a misleading picture of the safety of drugs to the older consumer. Indeed, the NSAIDs represent a glaring example of the contradiction between the promise and the reality of drug-taking in old age. The adverts are built around slogans which emphasise 'success', 'convenience' and 'simplicity'. The underlying reality may be more complex and may justify greater caution. Thus, research by Somerville et al. (1986) has related the use of NSAIDs to an increased risk of hospital admission with a bleeding peptic ulcer. The authors suggest that, if the findings from their Nottingham study were generally applicable to the UK population, there might be about 2000 cases of bleeding induced each year with, given a death rate of 10 per cent, about 200 deaths.

The researchers conclude:

> That such calculations are not fanciful is suggested by trends in admission rates of patients with perforated ulcer and the mortality from ulcer. The likelihood is that NSAIDs have an equivalent propensity to cause bleeding and perforation and although perforation rates have been falling in the past twenty five years in younger people, they have fallen little if at all in elderly men, but have risen in elderly women in a period when NSAID prescribing has become increasingly prevalent. The differential changes in perforation and mortality rates in men and women suggest that an association with anti-inflammatory drug use is not the simple and complete explanation. Nevertheless NSAID use is likely to be important, and measures to reduce the frequency and dose of NSAIDs in older people seem desirable (Somerville et al., 1986, p.464).

A Culture of Unsafety

The major difficulty we have to consider, given the above observations, is whether conventional advertising should be used as a medium of information where serious issues concerned with illness and disease are concerned. As with non-medical advertisements, what dominates the presentation is the initial claim or assertion. Thus the advertising for ketoprofen (brand name Oruvail) asks: 'Which anti-arthritic delivers success like this?' Underneath in large print are the figures 81 per cent and further down - in much smaller lettering - the note 'In a recent multi-centre trial over 12 weeks, a satisfactory response was obtained in 81 per cent of patients.' Without knowing more about the nature of the 'satisfactory response' or, indeed, the methodology of the trial, the claim is impossible to evaluate. However, its value is in projecting, in colourful and sensational terms, the superiority of the particular brand of drug. In some cases the claims made for drugs may be highly dubious. Thus, the manufacturers of dipyridamole (brand name Persantin), a drug on which the NHS spends some £5 million a year, were accused of making misleading claims about its value. Advertisements claimed that the drug could prevent heart attacks and strokes. However, two pharmacologists have concluded that there is no evidence to support this claim, and that it is little more effective than aspirin in preventing thrombosis (Drug and Therapeutics Bulletin, April 6 1984).

In May 1985 a number of companies were censured by the code of practice committee of the Association of the British Pharmaceutical Industry (ABPI). Glaxo, for example, was criticised for generating unjustified publicity in the lay press about its ulcer drug Zantac; Hoechst made unsubstantiated claims for its blood pressure drug Arelix; and Smith Laboratories were judged to have promoted an unlicensed painkiller in such a way as to have brought 'discredit on the industry'.

Tiaprofenic acid (brand name Surgam) was another NSAID to run into trouble, after an intensive advertising campaign in 1982 (the drug was billed as heralding: 'A move closer to the ideal in arthritis'). In this campaign, considerable emphasis was put on the ability of the drug to provide 'gastric protection'. If this had been the case, a major advance would have been made in the treatment for arthritis, given that traditional painkilling anti-inflammatory drugs (like aspirin and ibuprofen) can damage the digestive system and cause internal bleeding. However, the data sheet information, produced at the end of the advertisement, appeared to contradict the theme of 'gastric protection', cautioning use with patients 'with a history of peptic ulceration, severe renal or hepatic insufficiency, asthma or previous sensitivity to aspirin or other NSAID agents'. Moreover, 'gastric intestinal upsets' were accepted as one of the side effects of the drug. The discrepancy between the slogan and the potential impact of the drug caused the independent <u>Drug and Therapeutics Bulletin</u> to assert:

> The extravagant early promotion of Surgam, which might have endangered patients, faintly echoes that of benoxaprofen. These two examples should suffice to demonstrate the need for some surveillance of promotional claims. It is difficult to see how the CSM can decline this responsibility (<u>Drug and Therapeutics Bulletin</u>, 1 July 1983, p.50).

As a result of this criticism, the company substituted 'tolerance in the stomach' for the more controversial claim of 'gastric protection'.[9]

The Surgam case illustrates some general issues connected with advertising. A close analogy can be drawn with the problems surrounding cigarette advertising. In this instance, the bulk of the area contained by the publicity is given over to a positive sell for a particular brand of cigarette. Underneath, however, is the cautionary tale that the product may actually endanger your health. Drug advertising uses a very similar ploy. Prescribing information is typically present at the end of the advert, usually in very small type. This is often the case even with drugs known to exert harmful effects on groups such as older people. Thus, considerable data are available on the problems associated with anti-depressants when prescribed for older people. Prescribing information for one such drug, alpraxolam (brand name Zanex), informs the doctor that elderly people are particularly sensistive to its effects. After listing a number of contraindications, warnings, etc., the advert concludes: 'The elderly are particularly liable to experience these symptoms together with confusion, especially if organic brain symptoms are present.' The ABPI's code of practice indicates that this kind of information should be given clearly. However, in the case of the alpraxolam advert, prescribing information is presented in words one millimetre high, and compressed into 26 sentences just 6 and a half inches long. Two pharmacologists at St.George's Hospital in London asked 18 doctors to read the small print in this advert. They reported that: 'Three could not read the print and were not prepared to continue with it, three continued with the help of a magnifying lens, and one struggled through using a ruler to follow the lines.' The researchers concluded that: 'By their abuse of small print some pharmaceutical companies are ignoring advertising regulations and are making a mockery of the idea that advertisements should inform doctors about unwanted as well as wanted side effects' (Collier and New, 1984).

Similar criticism can be made of the advertising for zimeldine (brand name Zelmid), another anti-depressant drug, which was withdrawn from the UK market in November 1983 after reports of four deaths and 330 people experiencing side effects. The drug had shown particular promise in use with older people. Unfortunately, a small number proved particularly sensitive to the drug, and there was no way of determining which patients would suffer damaging side effects. Advertising had focused on the name Zelmid, this being printed in white against a black background and repeated in sufficient numbers to form a large square. Running through the print was a representation of a flash of lightning and underneath the slogan 'strikingly free from anti-depressant daytime sedation'. Of particular interest, however, is that the prescribing information section adopted a similar format, the advert being broken up by three lines of purple, describing where the drug offered advantages different from other products (or its differences) in comparison to other products. The general impact of the advert was to obscure any cautionary points it contained. In fact, buried half-way down the page, the alert and clear-sighted reader could find the note that: 'As a general principle, elderly and debilitated patients should be carefully monitored during therapy with anti-depressants, including Zelmid.' This warning certainly deserved a clearer presentation than was actually given, and it is difficult to see how it could pass any reasonable code of advertising standards.

Another example of prescribing information being presented in a way which is contrary to the interests of older people can be found with the drug indomethacin (brand name Indocid-R), a well-established NSAID. Up to early 1983, advertising for this drug carried a detailed summary (of approximately 1300 words) of the data sheet information. Buried within these data (and not highlighted to any extent) was the crucial information that: 'Indocid should be used with particular care in the older patient who may be more prone to adverse reactions.' This information was presented in the least helpful way to the doctor and was likely to be missed unless he or she was prepared to wade through the small print.

Conclusion

The promotional activities of many drug firms contrast somewhat unfavourably with the need for caution when introducing new drugs to older people. Indeed, in cases such as those illustrated by Opren (and other NSAIDs) the lucrative nature of the market often leads to premature and unjustifiable claims being made in relation to both safety and efficacy. This situation is further exacerbated by weaknesses in the professional care and support received by older people. In fact, as we shall argue in Chapter 4, it was the limitations of this support which was to give such a powerful presence to the drug companies in treatment strategies for older people. In the 1950s and 1960s the growth of the pharmaceutical companies went hand-in-hand with an ageing population. The enormous advances made by the pharmaceutical industry became influential in the determination of the medical construction of ageing - a development aided by the weaknesses in state controls and the limited influence of clinical pharmacology within primary care settings. In the next chapter we shall investigate the formation of the medical response to ageing, following the emergence of both geriatrics and the care of the elderly in general practice.

Footnotes

1. Criticisms of the CSM have been raised in articles by Shulman (1983b), Adams (1984) and Collier (1985).
2. The following section on benoxaprofen draws upon Phillipson, C. (1983); see also, Shulman, J. (1983a).
3. By July 1985 health ministers and the CSM were being sued by 900 patients who said they had been damaged by benoxaprofen (Guardian, 23 July 1985).
4. See Coleman's (1974) account of the media promotion of naproxen (another NSAID) which has parallels with the benoxaprofen case.
5. The relationship between parent companies and their subsidiaries is discussed in the Drug and Therapeutics Bulletin, 21, (20), 1983.
6. We are grateful to Candy Norris, Pharmacist, Hollymoor Hospital, Birmingham, for providing background

information about piroxicam.   See also the report in the Observer, 26 January 1986.

7.   See the Guardian, 14 and 15 March 1986.

8.   In the British context, the Drug and Therapeutics Bulletin, published by the Consumers Association, is an important exception.

9.   The manufacturers of Surgam were committed for trial in December 1985 on 10 charges involving advertising for tiaprofenic acid (Surgam).

Chapter 4

OLDER PEOPLE AND GERIATRIC MEDICINE

Introduction

This chapter will review the extent to which the practice and organisation of medicine has contributed, directly or indirectly, to the drug problems faced by older people. We shall consider how a range of factors - economic, demographic, cultural and educational - may have resulted in doctors being under-prepared for the impact of an ageing population, and vulnerable to pressures from drug companies. The chapter will review the development of geriatric medicine in Britain and abroad; it will also examine the pressures faced by general practitioners working in the community. Particular attention will be given to the question of 'medical dependency' and the impact this has had on older people. Finally, the chapter will consider a number of issues affecting older women in their relationship with doctors.

The Development of Geriatric Medicine

The link between medicine and older people is relatively recent. As late as the nineteenth century, few elderly people would have regular contact with a doctor, those who were very rich or very ill being the main exceptions (Stearns, 1977). For the physician, there were few guidelines regarding the care of his elderly patient. Most doctors prescribed - if they prescribed at all - the same as they would for younger people. In general, though, there was much pessimism about the value of medical intervention. According to the American historian Carol Haber: 'The weakness of the old was not considered a state amenable to cure. Instead, physicians believed that this was the essential irremediable quality of growing old' (Haber (C.), 1983, p.50). However, during the nineteenth century, specialist texts on ageing began to emerge. Innovation in therapy was particularly marked in Russia and the United States, closely followed by Germany, Britain and France. What developed in this period was the idea, elaborated in a classic text by Charcot (1882), that the diseases of old age required specialised investigation and analysis. Haber summarises the implications of this view as follows:

> He [the physician] could no longer assume that a single disease would have the same symptoms in all his patients, nor could he rely upon a unified therapeutic regimen. Disease categorization, based on the pathological transformation of tissues, necessitated a clear understanding of the normal and abnormal conditions for each stage of existence. The doctor who attempted to return senile tissue to its adolescent state would be truly foolhardy, if not indeed destructive. The elderly needed to be treated by standards that conformed to their own stage of life ... Here lay the basis for a specialization in the diseases of old age. The physician was required to know what ailments plagued the elderly, their physiological and anatomical basis, and the best - if any - method of treatment (Haber (C.), 1983, p.61).

The term 'geriatrics' was coined in 1909 by I.L. Nascher, in an article in the New York Medical Journal. Nascher carried out major work in the area of old age, writing one of the first handbooks on geriatrics. However, Achenbaum (1979) describes how his work met with considerable resistance, and that finding a firm willing to publish his research proved difficult. As late as 1926, Nascher admitted that he knew of no other scientist who described him or herself as a full-time geriatrician.

At the level of gerontological research there were important developments in the inter-war period, with the establishment of journals, the founding of gerontological institutes, and an increasing variety of scientific books and monographs (Howell, 1950; Cole, 1984; Amann, 1984). Yet the American historian Andrew Achenbaum (1979), suggests that the prevailing view of the 1920s and 1930s was that old age was a time of decrepitude, and that this was confirmed in the medical research of the period. This argument, however, ignores one of the most remarkable features of early twentieth century medical and health education literature, namely, its therapeutic optimism that old age could somehow be controlled and managed and that longevity was both possible and desirable.

Underpinning this medical movement was a change in popular thinking about the relative chances of survival. Traces of this can be found from a much earlier period. John McManners, for example, in his study of attitudes towards death in eighteenth century France, notes the psychological change which took place from the second half of the century. He writes:

> Before they knew for sure that the pattern of mortality
> was improving, some of the affluent minority were
> abandoning fatalism about growing old and dying.
> Against logic, they wanted to live longer, and they were
> discovering the logic to insist on enjoying life and being
> useful at a greater age (McManners, 1985, p.84).

What happened in the nineteenth and early twentieth centuries, was the diffusion of this sensibility to the expanding middle classes. With this change in popular thinking - which surely needs better documentation - came a flood of literature exploring how a healthy old age could be achieved. Cornaro's (1894) How to Regain Health and Live 100 Years By One Who Did It is an early example; however, it was soon followed by numerous texts, written by physicians, nutritionists, and exercise enthusiasts, identifying the way forward for a new generation of affluent elders.

The titles of these publications reflect the change in thinking: Outwitting Old Age (Asaker, 1926); Outwitting Middle Age (Ramus, 1926); Old Age Deferred (Lorand, 1910; Hollander, 1933); Grow Old and Stay Young (Dane, 1930); Live Longer and Be Happy (Barker, 1936). Some of these books were clearly aimed at the popular end of the market. Examples here would be Caprio and Grant's (1937) Why Grow Old? A guide-book for the man who seeks to remain physically and mentally young; and a British publication called Every Woman's Doctor Book (1934), which included a section on how to achieve 'A Healthy Old Age'.

Now it must be admitted that some of the recommendations in these books call to mind the old joke about doctors killing more than they cure. Hollander, a British physician and author of Old Age Deferred, was an enthusiast of the work of Voronoff who, pursuing the theme of rejuvenation in old age, had experimented with a number of grafting techniques involving the sexual glands of animals. According to Hollander:

> One of Voronoff's most striking cases was that of an old
> ram of twelve years - nearly the ram age limit - who was
> so senile and decrepit that he could hardly walk.
> Voronoff grafted into this old worn-out ram a sex gland
> from a two-year-old animal. A few months later the old
> ram was to all appearances a robust, virile, and splendid
> animal ... To leave no doubt as to cause and effect,
> Voronoff removed from the rejuvenated ram the gland
> grafts. The animal quickly lost its renewed youth and
> again became senile and decrepit. Once more Voronoff
> grafted new gland tissues, and, for the second time, the

senile ram became rejuvenated as completely as before (Hollander, 1933, p.67 and p.68).

Hollander also cites the work of Voronoff's colleague, a Dr. Steinach, whose grafting of sex glands onto human beings had less fortunate results: ' ... as in the notorious case of a German patient who, six months after being operated upon by Steinach, died in an asylum; and the similar case of an Englishman who arranged to deliver a lecture at the Albert Hall in London, on 'How I was made twenty years younger,' but died the day before that fixed for the lecture (presumably from heart disease)' (Hollander, 1933, p.65). Undeterred, Hollander comments: 'Further experiments and a longer period of observation are necessary before we can accept Steinach's results without reserve; but it must be acknowledged that they are perfectly reasonable, and that they follow as a logical sequence of many years' observation and experiments in this field' (Hollander, 1933, p.66).

At the same time, running through the literature of the early twentieth century were some important recommendations in the area of health education. Indeed, many of the texts pre-figured the health education movement of the 1980s, identifying the role of nutritional factors in enhancing life expectancy, and stressing the importance of physical fitness for older people (Lorand, 1910; Watson, 1913; Jeffery, 1939; Stieglitz, 1949; Gumpert, 1950).

Much of this literature was, it must be stressed, aimed at the affluent middle or upper class. For the working class elderly, however, there remained a significant gap between medical theory and practice. Inside the poor law infirmaries, conditions were often degrading (see below), with little attempt at rehabilitation. A restraining factor on the growth of geriatric medicine was the preoccupation in the 1920s and 1930s with the declining birth rate and the 'menace of under-population' (Branson and Heinemann, 1971, p.164). In this context, the health needs of the elderly were seen to be of minor importance compared with the health of children (Hobson, 1956). A Political and Economic Planning (PEP) report, completed in the late 1930s, which reviewed the state of Britain's health, managed to ignore entirely the question of the elderly (Herbert, 1939). Peter Stearns (1977) notes a similar situation in relation to France, where the decline in the birth rate encouraged even greater concentration on child-bearing and paediatrics.

The evidence suggests, in fact, two contrasting experiences in the period under discussion: first, the beginning of a debate about the medical basis for a healthy old age; secondly, the impoverished state of medical care for the bulk of elderly people. For our purposes, however, what is important is the radical change fostered by the impact of war and the ensuing labour shortages. These political and economic developments were to create new pressures for a proper medical service for old age. But whereas nutrition, exercise and other preventive factors were considered to be central in the 1920s and 1930s, they were to be overshadowed in the decades after the war. In their place, the role of drugs became a focal point in the medical construction of old age.

The Post-war Period

The late 1940s and early 1950s saw an upsurge of interest in the medical care of the elderly.[1] In the case of Britain, a number of factors influenced debates in this period. First, the idea of rehabilitation had been enhanced by the economic pressures during and immediately after the war. Trevor Howells notes how the need for 'employing older workers in the farms, the factories and the offices made the study of later life an urgent and vital necessity' (Howell, 1950, p.133). Labour shortages in the early 1950s meant that older people were encouraged to remain as full or part-time workers. This economic context may have helped to support the case of those arguing for more effective rehabilitation work amongst older people. MacIntyre (1977) notes the views of the Phillips Committee, who reported in 1954 on the financial implications of an ageing population. The report welcomed the rehabilitative approach ' ... both for the improvement it promises in health and happiness and for the relief to the heavy cost of looking after large numbers of chronic sick' (cited by MacIntyre, 1977, p.53).

Secondly, wartime conditions had themselves led, through the Emergency Medical Service, to a 're-discovery of the plight of the chronically ill aged in under-served and under-resourced municipal hospitals and infirmaries' (Carboni, 1982, p.76; see also Means and Smith, 1985). Thirdly, the development of the National Health Service provided financial and administrative support for the growth of geriatric medicine (Brocklehurst, 1978). Applicants for new consultant posts were also available. Carboni (1982), for example, notes the return to Britain of large numbers of consultants who were seeking new positions, but who faced a shortage of consultancies in the traditional medical specialties.

The immediate antecedents of British geriatrics can be found in the work of Dr. Marjory Warren at the West Middlesex Hospital in the 1930s. She had assumed responsibility for clinical care of the chronically sick in what was then a large poor law infirmary. Trevor Howell (himself a key figure in the development of British geriatric medicine) describes the infirmary in the following way:

The walls of the infirmary were all painted in shades of chocolate and dark green. The electric lighting was poor, giving little illumination to those wanting to read. Each ward contained an ill-assorted mixture of cases in its beds. Some were relatively healthy; others were sick and needed treatment ... Marjory Warren was given the task of reorganizing [the wards] ... She began by examining every patient and attempting to establish an adequate diagnosis. The healthy were separated from the sick. The young were taken away from wards full of old people. Thorough medical treatment was instituted and arrangements for discharge were made for those who did not require hospital attention and facilities. She next made a spirited attack on the gloomy surroundings which had depressed the patients under her care. Beds were now repainted in light pastel shades, yellow, green or blue. Walls were coloured cream. Better lighting was installed and unnecessary communicating doors were removed to make archways, creating large airy spaces. Modern lockers were obtained to give the patients a suitable place to keep their belongings. Bright red top blankets, light-coloured bedspreads and patterned screen curtains made the wards look cheerful. As the morale of the patients improved, they were encouraged to become more active. Many were got out of bed for the first time in years and allowed to sit in comfortable armchairs. Since many of the old folk were suffering from 'strokes' Dr Warren evolved a series of remedial exercises to aid their mobilization, to teach them to stand and encourage them to walk (Howell, 1976, p.445).

Another important figure was Lionel Cosin, medical superintendent at Orsell in Essex. Cosin, in an interview, gives the following account of the impact of his work treating elderly people with fractured hips:

When we started treating these patients and rehabilitating them physically ... we were staggered to find these patients, who had been defined by the local GPs as the chronically ill and irremediably sick, getting up and going home in two or three or four weeks (cited in Carboni, 1982, p.77).

Cosin, in fact, found that with active treatment 37 per cent of the elderly patients admitted could be discharged and 14 per cent rendered ambulant and accommodated in long-stay annexes (Morton, 1956). Amulree described the 'startling' effect of rehabilitation on long stay patients: 'the improvement in their physical condition being accompanied by an equal improvement in their mental state' (Amulree, 1951, p.41).
Underpinning these reforms in institutional care were changes in popular thinking about the possibilities for

achieving a healthy old age. People - the middle classes especially - continued their challenge to the fatalism which was typically attached to growing old. With the rise in membership of occupational pension schemes, the attraction of a lengthier retirement became clear. Retirement preparation courses, developed in Britain and America from the early 1950s, spelt out detailed advice on how to secure a healthy and financially secure old age (Phillipson, 1981). Handbooks on retirement started to be published from this period (see, for example, Chisholm, 1954). Guidebooks on how to handle health problems were also popular: Stieglitz's (1949) The Second Forty Years being a notable example. And middle class people themselves wrote books about how they had tackled and surmounted illnesses in later life: John Parr's (1951) How I Cured My Duodenal Ulcer and Eve Orme's (1955) My Fight Against Osteoarthritis being two such examples.

But behind these changes lay a genuine concern about the adequacy of existing therapies. Certainly, there was a quiet desperation faced by many who experienced illness in later life. One purchaser of Eve Orme's book wrote a dedication which expresses, in just a few words, this sense of despair: 'To my darling, in the hope that this book may help you, as I, alas, cannot.' As this suggests, who to turn to must have been a difficult dilemma for many in this post-war period, with constraints operating both on geriatric medicine and primary health care.

The Limitations of Medical Care

Despite the many initiatives in respect of institutional care, the 1950s and 1960s saw a protracted struggle by geriatricians for a larger share of research and nursing resources. Honigsbaum (1979) argues that conditions for the chronic sick actually worsened after 1948, with reactionary attitudes spreading from the voluntary sector to the hospital world as a whole. The buildings housing older people were invariably obsolete, and were only marginally improved, given the stagnation in hospital construction in the 1950s (Lindsey, 1962; Iliffe, 1983).

Part of the problem lay in attitudes towards demographic trends. Anxieties about the future size and composition of the population were expressed in reports from Political and Economic Planning (1948) and the Royal Commission on Population (1949). Both of these reports warned of economic difficulties due to a dip in the birth rate and the social pressures arising from more very elderly people (Phillipson, 1982).

As in the pre-war period, this demographic debate reinforced priorities in areas such as paediatrics. Armstrong summarises the success of the latter as follows:

Paediatricians, despite their smaller numbers in the NHS, rapidly established departments in all medical schools, a recognised place in the curriculum, a separate higher examination and high status. In contrast the very idea of geriatrics remained an essentially contested concept (Armstrong, 1981, p.253).

In some respects, the idea of rehabilitation was itself a challenge to the medical orthodoxy. Geriatric medicine met, according to Ivor Felstein, 'with heavy opposition from hospital colleagues in the medical wards, who could not see the value of spending time, money, energy or bed space on redundant senior members of the community' (Felstein, 1969, p.15). As late as 1972, the Annual Report of the Hospital Advisory Service reported comments from senior physicians along the lines of 'geriatricians are undesirable', and that 'medical patients should not be contaminated with geriatric patients' (cited in Bosanquet, 1978, p.131). One study in the 1970s found that medical students were less interested in elderly people at the end of their clinical training than at the beginning. A survey by Williamson found only one GP in three to be particularly interested in elderly patients or obtaining any job satisfaction from this part of their work (Mind, 1979, p.47).

There has, none the less, been a steady expansion in the number of consultant posts in geriatric medicine: the figure in 1981 was 390. However, Bernard Isaacs notes that, although impressive, this figure is still not enough, and that recruitment remains difficult. He writes:

Only a tiny proportion of recent graduates rate geriatric medicine as their career choice. This is not in itself surprising, since at that early stage of their career most young doctors seek general medical experience; and an interest in the elderly may not develop until a later stage. Any upsurge of interest in the elderly is likely to be discouraged by contemplation of the poor facilities and enormous work loads in geriatric departments; by the exclusion of many geriatric departments from general hospitals; by the relatively poor material rewards of the specialty; and, not least, by the derision and incredulity of well-meaning friends (Isaacs, 1981, p.149).

This depressing picture seems unlikely to have altered, given the constraints on health expenditure through the early 1980s (Iliffe, 1985; British Medical Association, 1986).

Problems within the institutional sector have spilled over to the community itself. Deficiencies in both medical training and availability of specialist help inevitably affected the work of the general practitioner. Population trends were gradually changing (drastically in some geographical areas) the composition of caseloads. Taking the national figures, those aged 75 plus increased from 920,000 in 1931, to 1,700,000 in 1951, reaching 3 million by 1981; amongst those 85 plus, the figures were 108,000 (1931) and 552,000 (1981).

To cope with this increase, official policy from the late 1950s gave increasing emphasis to the idea of 'community care'. Thus in 1958 the Minister of Health stated that the 'underlying principle of our services for the old should be this: that the best place for old people is in their own homes, with help from the home services if need be' (Townsend, 1964, p.196). The Hospital Plan (Ministry of Health, 1962, p.9) was said officially to rest on the expansion of community care services for its success. The Phillips Committee, in 1954, supported the case for 'active medical treatment followed by domiciliary care in the community' (cited in MacIntyre, 1977, p.54).

In practice, this new philosophy confronted formidable obstacles. Legislative support for domiciliary services - home helps, meals on wheels, etc. - was slow to emerge (MacIntyre, 1977). Services such as health visiting and district nursing were only just beginning to re-orientate themselves away from their traditional role - which had, historically, been the care of children and mothers. Health visiting, in fact, has never fully accepted work with older people, particularly as regards activity in the area of primary prevention and health education (Phillipson and Strang, 1984). Similarly, general practitioners, in line with the demographic priorities, expanded their work in antenatal care - helped by financial incentives (Oakley, 1984). In contrast, work with older people was approached with less enthusiasm, partly because it was also considered to be much less remunerative.

Williamson et al.'s (1964) study of 'unreported needs' amongst the elderly opened a debate about the need to develop an effective preventive service for older people. The researchers argued that:

... most old people do not report their complaints to their doctors until the condition is advanced. Thus a general practitioner service based on the self-reporting of illness is likely to be seriously handicapped in meeting the needs of old people. It might be argued that many of the unknown disabilities we detected are degenerative and progressive, and therefore not amenable to curative measures. This is unjustifiably pessimistic; preventive medicine is at least as important in old age as it is earlier in life, and there are few conditions in old people which medical and social measures, applied soon enough, will not help. Indeed in many of these degenerative states, further progress of disability can be arrested or at least slowed down (Williamson et al., 1964, p.1120).

Williamson et al. (1964) pressed for health visitors to do periodic visiting to the homes of old people and to carry out screening on behalf of general practitioners. This was accepted by some health visitors but, in general, as observed above, the profession was lukewarm about work with the elderly; indeed, the proportion of older people in the caseloads of health visitors declined slightly during the 1970s.

Finally, a continuing problem has been the variations in care received by the elderly from general practitioners. This seems particularly the case in respect of the GP's role as a gatekeeper to other services, and his or her willingness to work with health visitors, social workers and other professional carers (Phillipson and Strang, 1984; Wilkin, 1983).

The Golden Age of Drugs

Despite the obstacles listed above, the needs of older people still had to be serviced by the medical profession. In responding to these needs, however, the GP or consultant did have one powerful ally, namely, the pharmaceutical companies. Faced with the mental distress arising from widowhood or the range of chronic conditions affecting older people, drugs were to emerge as a dominant method of treatment. Drugs for the elderly became, in fact, a boom industry from the 1960s onwards. At the same time, the drug companies had themselves entered a period of accelerated expansion.

In the post-war era, effective medicines multiplied at an unparalleled rate (Midlands Bank Review, 1985). Inside the NHS, proprietary drugs grew in importance: from around one-fifth of all prescriptions in 1950, to nearly half just seven years later. The yearly NHS drugs bill grew at an increasingly faster rate, approaching £2000 million by the mid-1980s. Underpinning the drugs boom was the demand for tranquillisers (from the mid-60s onwards), antihypertensives (from the mid to late 60s), and NSAIDs (from the mid-70s). By the 1970s, 1 in 5 of all elderly people were taking 3 or more medicines daily; 1 in 10 were taking four or more.

The drug companies undoubtedly flourished in the market provided by an expanding elderly population. Some of this expansion reflects the greater prevalence of disabling conditions which accompanies an ageing population. However, it is also possible to trace other factors which have contributed to this growth.

First, drugs emerged as the treatment of 'first choice' partly through the absence of viable alternatives. There was, for example, very limited awareness of the role of preventive medicine (perhaps even less than in the inter-war period), and doctors were given little encouragement to think beyond what the drug companies might be offering. Some geriatricians and GPs did carry out important work in the area of prevention and health education. Ferguson Anderson and his colleague Nairn Cowan are two obvious examples. Anderson was active in pre-retirement education and helped to form, in 1958, the Glasgow Retirement Council (the first association of its kind in Great Britain).[2] He also developed, with Cowan, screening facilities for older men and women, at the Rutherglen Consultative Health Centre (Anderson and Cowan, 1955). Yet this work had limited short- and medium-term influence. Very few health workers became interested in pre-retirement education, and health screening, particularly for middle-aged unskilled and semi-skilled workers, remains patchy and underdeveloped in many areas.

A second reason for the increasing importance of drugs was the fact that their danger for older people was consistently underplayed. General practitioners, particularly in the 1950s and 1960s, relied upon the drug companies for information about new medication (see Chapter 3). There is some evidence that this information was used rather more in conditions affecting older people; in other areas, the doctor relied upon his/her own training or neutral sources. Unfortunately, the drug companies almost certainly under-estimated the harmful effects of drugs on older people.

Thirdly, the very lack of facilities and resources was (and continues to be) a fact promoting the use of drugs. Moreover, the policy of community care, though attractive to those anxious to stimulate a move away from Victorian institutions, actually created new problems, given the failure to audit and control the prescribing of drugs. The end results were the numerous stories of 'drug hoarding', abuses of repeat prescribing, etc., which unfolded in the 1970s and 1980s (Tuft, 1982). Almost invariably it was older people who were cited in these stories. But the message - that professionals were themselves responsible for the problem and that the drug companies had the most to gain - was usually ignored.

Older People and the Practice of Medicine

So far we have indicated some general factors influencing the extent of drug use among older people. A contributory aspect, however, concerns the characteristics of medicine in our society. Over the past 30 years there has been a strengthening in the doctor's position as a person interpreting a range of medical, psychological and social dilemmas. Critics have spoken of the problem of 'medical dependency'. Porter, for example, observes that: 'In the world we have lost, people didn't become dependent upon doctors and their doses, because neither doctor nor the sick believed that medicine held all the answers to people's complaints' (Porter, 1984, p.88). Zola (1978), in a major critique of contemporary medicine, saw the profession as laying claim for responsibility for a range of illnesses and conditions, irrespective of whether an effective response was possible. However, medicine's 'claim to responsibility' for problems affecting older people has created a number of difficulties. Medical dependency has taken the form of a denial of older people's ability to manage and control their health problems in later life. Diagnostic skills, blood pressure control, home nursing, exercise and nutrition education programmes have all been seriously underdeveloped (Coppard, 1984; Savo, 1984). Doctors (and nurses) have rarely attempted properly to educate their patients, seemingly preferring the power which comes from controlling key items of knowledge. The result has been an elderly population vulnerable to the alluring claims of drug companies suggesting instant relief or cures for chronic diseases. In addition, medical dependency has fed into and has itself reinforced structural processes which confirm old age as a period of reduced power and self-esteem (Townsend, 1981). This is felt most acutely in client relationships in the health and social services. Lewis Coser characterises these relationships in the following way: 'The professional and [the client] ... belong to two basically different worlds ... and the asymmetry is not only of feelings and attitudes, it is also an asymmetry of power' (cited in Estes, 1979, p.25).

The hierarchical nature of care relations has been explored in a range of studies (Evers, 1982; Fairhurst, 1977; Webb and Hobdell, 1980). These have indicated the limited attention to the patient's own perspectives on his or her illness, together with the exclusion of patients and relatives from the decision-making process.

The unequal relationship between doctor and older patient has limited the understanding of each about the nature of growing old. Neither has been prepared for the realities of ageing. Doctors have rarely been prepared to submit themselves to an open dialogue about what medicine can or cannot offer. For older people, there has been a contradiction between, on the one hand, heightened expectations about the value of medical interventions and, on the other, pessimism about the possibility of improving physical and mental health problems. For both groups - doctors as well as the elderly - recourse to drugs may offer a useful device where some sort of action is needed. But the short-term comfort provided may come at the expense of long-term physical dependence and harmful side-effects.

Women and Prescribing

An additional area affecting patterns of prescribing concerns sex differences between the doctor and his or her patient. In fact, whilst men form the majority of GPs (six out of every seven GPs are male) and consultant geriatricians, the majority of their elderly patients will be women. This is because (a) two thirds of pensioners are women; (b) women are, according to the General Household Survey (OPCS, 1984), more likely than men to visit doctors; (c) they experience the greater morbidity associated with old age (Women's National Commission, 1984). This imbalance has further reinforced processes leading to social and medical dependency. Leeson and Gray (1978) argue that women's health problems tend to be denigrated by doctors, at all stages of the life cycle. However, women in middle and old age may experience more difficulties with their doctors, given the rise in consultation rates in later life. Barrett and Roberts (1978), in a study of the treatment by GPs of middle-aged women, have noted how doctor and patient accept stereotyped definitions of the problems facing women patients. They found that the GPs seemed to endorse the prevailing ideology regarding sex roles, viewing women as 'naturally' preoccupied with their home and family, and men 'naturally' more concerned with their occupational life. Barrett and Roberts suggested that these assumptions were: 'not merely reflected in the practice of medicine but [were] actively endorsed and sanctioned with medical authority' (Barrett and Roberts, 1978, p.44; see also Roberts, 1985).

Ideologies relating to sex roles are also important in old age. Thus doctors may be dismissive about the retirement problems of their female patients, assuming that the maintenance of a 'housework role' will prove sufficient interest. Those women who feel otherwise may be dismissed as 'neurotic' and 'unrealistic', their worries either being ignored or responded to with, for example, an anti-depressant drug.

Another important problem concerns the deference shown by women towards their GPs. This was highlighted in the study by Barrett and Roberts (1978, p.50), and they concluded that its effect was to leave undiscussed the real problems facing the patient. This problem may be particularly damaging in old age, where bereavement and the death of close friends may have complex emotional and psychological repercussions. Unfortunately, the patient may find it difficult to break from a long-established pattern of deference, developed with a particular doctor or practice. This passivity may actually be encouraged by the doctor, who may view the ideal patient as one who is 'passive, obedient and co-operative' (Stimson, 1974). In effect, the ideal person may be one who will be least questioning about drugs, their relevance or likely side effects.

Conclusion

This chapter has tried to show the range of influences which led to the popularity of drugs for older people. Amongst those identified were: the slow emergence of geriatric medicine; the child-care orientation of the general practitioner and community nursing service (complemented, of course, by a similar bias in social work - Rowlings, 1981; Black et al., 1984); the under-resourcing of domiciliary support; the encouragement of patient dependency; and the problems faced by women patients in their interaction with (predominantly) male doctors. These factors - exacerbated by the neglect of geriatrics and preventive gerontology in vocational training and continuing education - created a fertile ground for the drug industry to exert its influence.

Older people, in fact, have become the drug industry's 'most important customer' (Comfort, 1983, p.117). This is partly through medical need and genuine suffering, partly through a dearth of therapeutic alternatives (e.g. for depression and hypertension), and partly through sheer ignorance about what drugs can achieve. In addition, consumer demand, stimulated by a belief in the inevitability of old age, has been important in stimulating the use of drugs. But the growth of the industry has been underpinned by social processes and assumptions which encourage, first, the idea of medical dependency; secondly, the view of ageing as a physical and biological process of decrement and decline - the so-called biomedical model of ageing (Estes et al., 1984); thirdly, an establishment view of preventive geriatrics as an inferior branch of medicine. The conclusion must be that the medical and pharmaceutical complex has been a powerful force in the construction of ageing in the twentieth century. Its dominance has been assisted by a wider, cultural pessimism as regards ageing. Medical and lay beliefs have, in fact, shared an underlying symmetry in their perceptions about growing old. Both have operated within a framework of rejection; both have adopted models of change which ignore the variety and complexity of the ageing process, and the possibilities for growth and discovery, in addition to experiences of illness and loss. In contrast with this, the drug companies have been able to suggest that they hold, through their own endeavours, the answer to the medical and social 'crisis' wrought by an ageing population. True, many of their creations have been positive and beneficial: the companies themselves pour out tons of promotional material telling us that this is so. In contrast, however, we have been given fewer hand-outs on the problems and dangers - particularly as they apply to groups such as older people. In the next three chapters we examine in more detail the risks and benefits of drugs for older people.

Footnotes

1.   One aspect of this was the formation, in 1947, of the Medical Society for Care of the Elderly (later to be renamed the British Geriatric Society).   The Society was formed by Lord Amulree and Dr. Trevor Howell.

2.   For a brief history of the Glasgow (now Scottish) Retirement Council, see Phillipson and Strang (1983); see also Phillipson, 1981.   The most recent survey of pre-retirement provision is provided by Coleman (1982).

PART II: Experiences of Drug Use

Chapter 5

OLDER PEOPLE AND THE USE OF PSYCHOTROPIC DRUGS

Introduction

The psychotropics are the main category of mood-altering drugs prescribed by doctors; they include sedatives, stimulants, . tranquillisers and anti-depressant medications. Within the psychotropic group there is a bewildering multiplicity, many drugs having the same pharmacological actions. There is little clarification for the GP, at the sharp end of clinical practice, on the distinction between drugs and on their individual limitations. The GP is often confronted with a range of conflicting and exaggerated information from the drug companies; new drugs are introduced at a bewilderingly fast rate. Unfortunately, not only is the need for them uncertain, as many are very similar to products already on the market, but also the full spectrum of side effects has yet to be elucidated, and this may take at least 5-10 years for an individual drug. The vast variety of psychotropic drugs, the polished quality of the publicity for their use and the attendant creation of an unlimited market, amplifies the demand for drugs. It overwhelms the more critical scientific literature to which the doctor might become exposed, calling upon stamina, self-discipline and a background of thorough initial training to resist. However, resistance is one thing, providing alternative methods of treatment and management is another.

Prevalence of Drug Use

The issue of mass usage finds particular currency with the psychotropic drugs because of the ubiquitous nature of anxiety and bodily symptoms that stem from chronic degenerative diseases. The use of sedatives and minor tranquillisers has risen by two to three times in the last twenty years; this increase is especially marked in the case of older people. In a community survey of psychotropic drug use, Williams (1980) reported that 14 per cent of men and 22 per cent of women over the age of 65 years admitted to taking at least one psychotropic drug in the previous two weeks. In the age group 45-64, the figures were 9 per cent for men and 17 per cent for women. This is not just short-term but involves long-term use of drugs.

Research in the United States, by the National Institute of Drug Abuse, showed older people to consume disproportionate amounts of psychotropic drugs:

> ... in the case of Thorizine (a major tranquilizer), the sedatives, the non-barbiturate hypnotic, and three out of four of the barbiturate hypnotics, older people receive over one-fourth of all drug orders
> ... Despite the fact that the elderly are 11 per cent of the total population, they consume 21.2 per cent of all orders for Valium (minor tranquilizer), 23.4 per cent of all orders for Librium (minor tranquilizer), 30.4 per cent of all orders for Dalmane [flurazepam] (nonbarbiturate hypnotic), 21.1 per cent of all orders for Phenobarbital [phenobarbitone] (a sedative) (cited in Breen, 1982, p.80).

Widespread and heavy use of psychotropic drugs amongst the elderly has been confirmed worldwide in the developed countries. In Australia, for example, Chapman (1976) reported that although pensioners made up only 9 per cent of the population, they consumed 45 per cent of psychotropic drugs issued by the Australian National Health Service. In a study in Oxford by Skegg et al. (1977), all prescriptions issued to a population of about 40,000 people were studied. During one year, 53.8 per cent of all males and 65.7 per cent of all females had at least one form of drug dispensed. The proportion who received medicines increased with age and was higher among females of all ages. They found that psychotropic drugs were prescribed more often than any other group of drugs and accounted for almost one-fifth of all prescriptions.

From a survey of the use of psychotropic drugs in Finland (Riska and Klaukka, 1984), significantly more such drugs were taken in relation to increasing age (especially amongst women), the presence of chronic physical illness and the number of visits the patient made to the doctor. This research also found that those in the lowest income bracket were prescribed significantly more psychotropic drugs than those with higher incomes.

In a study sponsored by the DHSS of drug-taking habits of elderly people in different living situations, Wade and Finlayson (1983) found that psychotropic drugs were the most commonly taken drug. One-third of the elderly men and about half of the women took such drugs. These figures were then broken down according to the different sectors of care. There was considerable variation in the use of drugs in the main groups of medicines, the extremes showing most clearly with the psychotropics. Among patients in the care of community nurses, 18 per cent were taking a psychotropic drug; in the private nursing sector, however, the figure rose to 78 per cent. Many patients/residents were taking more than one drug at a time. This problem was most acute in the private nursing sector, with 21.1 per cent of residents taking two, and 3.5 per cent three psychotropic drugs in the 24 hours preceding the survey. These figures were substantially higher than for the hospital sector (6.7 per cent and 1.7 per cent respectively) despite the fact that the dependency levels of patients in hospitals and private nursing homes were broadly comparable.

For older people, these and other drugs inevitably produce mental impairment. According to Alex Comfort: 'For the non-demented person, serious mental impairment is intensely disturbing and in a sizeable proportion of cases where anxiety over this is a presenting symptom, the patient is on benzodiazepines, tricyclic antidepressants, digoxin, uncompensated diuretics or more than one of these. The intellectual impairment is genuine and the treatment is to stop the medication, when it will recover' (Comfort, 1982, p.160).

The Use of Minor Tranquillisers and Hypnotics

Hindmarsh (1981) has made extensive studies on the effects of psychotropic drugs on performance of everyday activities. He argues that sedation as a 'side effect' of anxiety treatment, as well as the residual hypnotic or sedative activity in the morning after taking sleep inducers, can also produce a deterioration in performance skills. Research findings in normal subjects show that many psychotropic drugs, including the benzodiazepines, have adverse effects on movements involving some element of skill. The drugs may thus be causative or contributory agents in accidents at home and when driving. One researcher notes that: 'All these effects may last many hours after single doses, persist through long-term administration, are potentiated by alcohol and other depressants and are more marked and longer lasting in the elderly' (Ashton, 1983, p.360).

Short-acting benzodiazepines are said to be less likely to cause 'hangovers' or cumulative effects. Yet a study by Betts and Birtle (1982) showed that temazepam, a relatively short-acting drug heavily prescribed as a hypnotic for older people, adversely affected driving performance even in non-elderly subjects 12 hours after a single night-time dose. Such effects are not restricted to psychotropic drugs and can occur with, for example, the NSAIDs, analgesics, and hypotensive agents (Ashton, 1983).

The measured effects on reaction time, following both

single-dose and repeated treatment with an extensive range of benzodiazepines (the commonly used minor tranquillisers), has been shown to be independent of the drug-handling characteristics of the drugs. Those with 'short half-lives' are just as potent in disrupting skilled performance as are those with longer elimination times. Improvement in the psychological condition of patients treated with psychotropic drugs can often be cancelled out if there are noticeable sedative effects which reduce the level of activity of the central nervous system and upset the equilibrium between sensory and motor systems.

Benzodiazepines (especially midazolam) are in fact used in premedication before surgery, because they have a useful effect of producing memory loss for some three hours or more after consumption. Hindmarsh suggests in fact that this memory loss is probably a reflection of the reduction in overall arousal within the central nervous system. He suggests that as complex sensorimotor performance (e.g. driving) is in part dependent on memory, drugs that produce memory loss are likely to interfere with the performance of intellectual tasks. This is especially the case with very elderly people.

Hindmarsh (1981) details the complexity surrounding many types of investigation into psychomotor function with psychotropic drugs, and the problems associated with interpreting the results of performance tests. However, it seems that any drug that has a sedative effect impairs psychomotor performance and memory-processing ability; further, they have a synergistic (multiplying) effect with other sedative drugs and alcohol. Subhan (1984) reports that whereas commonly used benzodiazepines such as diazepam and lorazepam may show no serious reduction of consciousness the drugs are likely to act upon the process of memory retention rather than registration or recall.

There is also a paradoxical effect which occasionally arises through the use of benzodiazepine drugs. Contrary to the expected calming effect, patients become tense, sleepless, antagonistic and prone to aggressive outbursts (British Medical Journal leader, 1975; Goldney, 1977; Edwards 1981). Such reports have shown the occurrence of disinhibition, loss of control and aggression - especially when people are grouped together - being more common than is generally realised. These results suggest that older people in overcrowded residential settings may be particularly vulnerable to such side effects.

In the past there has been uncertainty as to whether benzodiazepines lead to weight loss or weight gain. Recently, in a double blind trial in 97 volunteers aged 40-68, Oswald and Adam found the benzodiazepines (nitrazepam and lormetazepam given at night) compared with placebo produced a small yet significant loss of body weight over a period of 32 weeks. Oswald and Adam point out that this weight loss should not be assumed to entail body fat: 'The muscle relaxant action or a small degree of lethargy, leading to less muscular work, and slight loss of body muscle over a period of months, provide one among other possible explanations' (Oswald and Adam, 1980, p.1040). Were this to be the case, the loss of further body muscle in an already frail elderly person could contribute to a loss of independent activity.

Sedatives provoke ataxia (unsteadiness) in the elderly (Edwards, 1981). The chances of falling and fracturing frail bones is enhanced amongst this age group. A survey of femoral fractures in patients aged over 65 by the Macdonalds (1977) found that, of 390 patients with such fractures, nearly all had been caused by nocturnal falls when most of the patients were taking barbiturate hypnotics. They also found that the barbiturates themselves were also strongly associated with a history of frequent falls. They went on to report that among new outpatients at a geriatric clinic, falls or episodes of dizziness were a reason for referral in over 85 per cent of patients taking barbiturates, but in less than one quarter of patients not on these drugs.

Confusion in older people sometimes progressing to a pseudodementia (dementia-like picture) has been described with long-term barbiturate use (Rudd, 1972) and more significantly long-term nitrazepam (Mogadon) use (Evans, 1972). The Macdonalds (1977) further reported that over half the patients weaned off barbiturates in hospital improved their mental status questionnaire (MSQ) score by 3 points or more. The MSQ measures orientation on a 0-17 point scale. In recording this improvement in score from that on admission to that on discharge by 3 points or more they emphasised that this could well mean the difference between independence and institutional care.

They were further disconcerted that over 40 per cent of old people referred to a geriatric outpatient service in Nottingham in 1973 were on barbiturates, despite long-standing warnings on the dangers of barbiturates in this age group; by 1976 this figure had actually risen to over 50 per cent. Since the mid-1970s there has been a slow overall decline in the taking of barbiturates, though other evidence points to a residual persistence by some doctors in their use (Wade et al., 1983). It suggests that night sedation for older people, with the high level of repeat prescriptions, has become a self-perpetuating feature of medical practice.

The Use of the Major Tranquillisers (Neuroleptics)

Neuroleptics are given to older people for their specifically antipsychotic effects in, for example, schizophrenia and in psychotic states of extreme excitement and elation. They are also used, although this is more problematic, for their non-specific effects upon disturbed behaviour. Over-reliance on these powerful drugs brings forth the accusation that they are used as a 'chemical strait-jacket'. Their use for vociferous or uncooperative residents in homes for the elderly undoubtedly requires serious questioning (American Psychiatric Association, 1980; Barnes et al., 1982).

Neuroleptics (as well as benzodiazepine drugs) can also have the paradoxical effects of increasing anxiety and aggression (Rice and Arie, 1981). Their use - especially long-term - should be curtailed amongst older people because of the risk of a wide range of adverse side-effects. They seriously impair movement when administered over a long period, producing stiffness and tremor as in Parkinson's disease, as well as restless 'jitters' and involuntary movements distorting the face, mouth and tongue. All these are produced significantly more amongst older people (Barnes, 1984), who may already have movement problems. Anti-parkinsonian drugs can be given to reduce these side effects, though should these drugs be increased to control persistent abnormal movements they can make some of the movements worse, in particular those distorting the face, mouth and tongue (tardive dyskinesia).

Age is the major variable influencing both prevalence and severity of tardive dyskinesia (Kane and Smith, 1982; Barnes et al., 1983). The older the patient when starting neuroleptic drug treatment the more rapidly the condition develops. For drug-induced movement disorders like tardive dyskinesia and parkinsonism, Barnes states that, 'The only effective pharmacological manoeuvre is withdrawal of the provoking anti-psychotic (neuroleptic) drug' (Barnes, 1984, p.733). The addition of anti-parkinsonian agents in the elderly to counteract the effect of the neuroleptic can be disappointing. They themselves can produce confusion, restlessness, hallucinations, outbursts of delirious shouting and impaired memory (Drug and Therapeutics Bulletin, 1984). This in turn may induce the doctor to prescribe more of the neuroleptic in a spiral of false therapeutic optimism.

There are many other important side effects amongst the neuroleptic drugs including loss of temperature control, sudden falls of blood pressure (leading to faints and falls), skin reactions, jaundice, drug interactions, weight gain and difficulties in sexual functioning (Kotin et al., 1976).

Neuroleptic drugs are often prescribed in residential homes on the basis of judgements about the behaviour of elderly residents, i.e. staff may seek to control 'unacceptable' behaviour with major tranquillisers. Ideas about acceptable behaviour vary, however, from home to home. Appropriate models for prescribing powerful anti-psychotic drugs, especially amongst frail older people, urgently need to be established.

In a survey of patterns of neuroleptic use among the

institutionalised elderly, Gilleard et al. (1983) observed marked variations between homes and between wards and hospitals. The survey was carried out among residents of local authority homes for the elderly and elderly patients in geriatric, psychogeriatric and general hospital wards in one of the London Boroughs. Out of an institutionalised population of 839,107, 13 per cent were found to be taking neuroleptic drugs. This concealed wide variations, although there was little overall difference in the level of neuroleptic use between residential homes and hospitals as a whole. Within both sectors, variation was considerable, ranging from 0 to 28 per cent in the different homes and from 0 to 43.5 per cent in the different hospital wards. Gilleard et al. found that for the total sample it was possible to derive a profile of the characteristics of the elderly institutionalised patient to whom neuroleptics are likely to be administered – namely, someone confused, partially in touch with his or her surroundings, weepy, never cheerful, disturbing to others at night and on concurrent doses of hypnotics.

Despite this marked variation in the use of neuroleptics between homes, the condition of the residents and their overall behavioural disturbance did not vary. There was a trend for the homes with higher levels of hypnotic use also to have higher levels of neuroleptic use. To account for the variation between homes Gilleard et al. concluded that factors relating to institutional practice, rather than residents' disabilities, play a significant role in determining the use of neuroleptics (see Chapter 7). In contrast, variations of neuroleptic drug use between hospital wards seemed to be significantly associated with variations in patient disabilities. He further questioned whether confusion made worse by neuroleptic drugs was actually recognised. In the absence of psychosis, the use of neuroleptics for elderly patients was postulated to serve institutional rather than individual needs.

A report by Fottrell et al. (1976) reviewed psychotropic medication in 200 randomly selected long-stay psychiatric patients. In over three-quarters an organic psychosis such as dementia or schizophrenia was diagnosed, half were aged 65 or more. In a careful follow-through study these patients' medication was altered or stopped and the patients later assessed by the same team after six months. They found that about half the patients on psychotropic drugs had been receiving unnecessary or excessive medication. Fottrell expressed concern at the absence of regular routine reviews of medication in these long-term patients and criticised the philosophy regarding medication, namely that of 'leave well enough alone'. Since there are few time-related standard dosages in psychiatry, the end result is that many elderly psychiatric patients, both within and outside hospital, remain on unnecessary or excessive medication for long periods.

Simple observations or subjective perceptions of those on

the major tranquillisers would confirm that finer levels of consciousness and alertness are severely blunted, especially as the dosage rises. Dosages of thioridazine (Melleril), a 'safer' neuroleptic for the elderly, of 25 mg three times a day (a dosage usually well tolerated in the younger patient) is, in anyone over 75, almost certain to produce marked inertia and drowsiness after long-term usage. Yet this dose is commonly given to older people in institutions. Neuroleptics can cause many other problems. Bliss (1981) found that neuroleptics were the most common cause of drug-induced illness necessitating admission and that most of the victims were older people. Most frequently, it was related to severe falls of blood pressure, drowsiness, confusion and parkinsonism.

Another heavily over-prescribed drug, without any clinical justification in older people, is prochlorperazine (Stemetil). This is a drug used to control the giddiness of Ménière's disease in younger people, but wittingly or unwittingly heavily promoted and prescribed for the ubiquitous symptom of giddiness in the elderly. Giddiness may stem from sudden falls of blood pressure which prochlorperazine itself readily induces, especially with older people! Stephen and Williamson (1984) reported on a survey of all new cases of parkinsonism referred to the department of geriatric medicine at the City Hospital, Edinburgh, over a two-year period. Ninety-five cases of parkinsonism were diagnosed: 48 (51 per cent) were associated with prescribed neuroleptic drugs. The commonest drug responsible was prochlorperazine (21 cases) and the second commonest was thioridazine (Melleril - 13 cases). The authors say that in none of the prochlorperazine cases was there any suggestion of a valid indication for the drug. They went on to urge extreme caution in the use of neuroleptics in the elderly.

Drug-induced parkinsonism is much commoner than most people have been led to believe (Williamson, 1984). After stopping the offending drug, Williamson writes that anti-parkinsonian drugs should not then be prescribed for twelve months because the features of drug-induced illness linger on for such a long time. Sometimes the features of parkinsonism are not obvious. The patient presents more with a lack of movement (akinetic parkinsonism), facial immobility and dribbling from the mouth. The condition may be mistaken for apathy or depression and should be suspected when an elderly patient mysteriously 'goes off her feet'. This type of parkinsonism may take weeks after the introduction of the neuroleptic to develop and go unrecognised for years.

The Value of Drug Treatment for Anxiety in the Elderly

Despite common clinical observations that responses to the various benzodiazepines differ considerably between individual patients, several well-conducted studies among large numbers of people have produced a general consensus as to the substantial clinical similarity of all benzodiazepines (Greenblatt and Shader, 1974; Kesson et al., 1976). This view has been upheld by the Committee for the Review of Medicines (CRM). Individual and unpredictable differences in kinetics (drug handling) largely explain the apparent variety of effects and side effects.

In addition, marketed dosage also explains the differing effects. Each benzodiazepine can act in the same patient as an anti-anxiety drug at lower dosage as well as a hypnotic at a higher dose. With older people, as we have previously mentioned, this distinction becomes more blurred because of delayed elimination and accumulation and because of the increased sensitivity at the site of action in the brain. As an example of this bonus for the drug companies, temazepam (Euhypnos), recently introduced in the UK as a hypnotic with a recommended dosage of 10 to 30 mg at bedtime, has been used in Italy for many years as an anxiolytic agent in 5 mg tablets, manufactured by the same firm.

The prescription of anti-anxiety and sedative drugs has at least doubled during the past twenty years. This increase rises with advancing age, especially amongst the very old in institutions (Wade et al., 1983). The steep rise with age is more marked in males than females, despite 70 per cent of all hypnotics actually being prescribed to females.

The problem of treating anxiety at any age, but especially amongst older people, is compounded by the lack of clarity in its classification as a clinical phenomenon, together with limitations in treatment strategies (Tyrer, 1984a). Much anxiety among older people is provoked by the constraints of their living environment and the sheer problem of coping in situations of poverty and bad housing (Phillipson and Walker, 1986). Loneliness and a long-standing anxious disposition are other common reasons why elderly patients visit their doctor; it has also been found that the chance of being prescribed a minor tranquilliser is related to the frequency of visits to the GP (Riska and Klaukka, 1984).

In the case of anxiety arising out of everyday stresses and crises, a major question-mark hangs over the value of treatment with sedative/tranquillising drugs. Without drugs, but with counselling help, the patient might cope with her anxiety or she might do something to avert the crisis. Given sedatives, she will do neither, but wait for the attack to subside. These drugs may reduce clinical anxiety, but are much less successful in preventing the anxiety attack or panic attack proper (Snaith 1983).

In some people, benzodiazepines produce a paradoxical increase in anxiety feelings (Parrott and Kentridge, 1982). This unwanted effect of unpleasant anxiety can also be a day-time consequence of night-time sedation, or simply the result of the cessation of treatment. Tyrer et al. reported that, even after the immediate withdrawal phenomena from benzodiazepines have passed, patients are more vulnerable to the stresses of life: 'Possibly because their coping mechanisms have become atrophied during their long period of drug therapy' (Tyrer et al., 1983, p.1406).

James (1978) questions whether anxiety in older people warrants drug intervention at all. Like many others before him, he says that sometimes a certain amount of worry is quite acceptable. If action is necessary, it is to do with the fact that anxiety is often triggered by other factors which demand positive intervention. Amongst older people this is often money, housing or health. James goes on to say that reassurance from the GP or appropriate social advice may be all that is needed. Reassurance about health worries is usually only successful if the patient is fully examined. Strong reassurance, he says, is better than a 'fist full of tranquillisers' (James, 1978, p.57).

Depressive Illness in the Elderly and Antidepressant Drugs

It has been estimated that one-third to one-half of all depressive illnesses occur in later life. Treatment in the short term is good, but over the long term depression can show high morbidity and a tendency to recur (Jacoby, 1981; Murphy, 1983).

Shepherd et al. (1966) found that when family doctors saw depressed elderly patients, sedatives and tranquillisers were the most frequently offered therapy. Such drugs only have a transient calming effect, with no resolution of the morbid depression; so that unfortunately, escalating dosage, polypharmacy, or long-term drug dependency may follow. In the true biological depressive illness (sometimes called psychotic or endogenous depression) an appropriate dosage schedule of antidepressant medication can lead to a remission. However, these drugs carry risks which are increased in the elderly because of altered drug handling and an enhanced sensitivity. Drug elimination is delayed, higher steady states including blood levels result, and in turn adverse effects are much more frequent and profound (Neis et al., 1977).

It is important to remember that true antidepressant drugs are not stimulants or euphoriants, having an immediate action on the individual. Their antidepressant effect does not appear for two to three weeks. The repeated claim that newer (much more expensive) antidepressant drugs act more quickly has not been substantiated. These particular drugs are, in addition, of no special value in 'treating' the elderly or others with intolerable social situations or unresolved problems associated with, for example, bereavement.

The common practice of giving a night sedative and even daytime sedation plus an antidepressant is unnecessary and

Psychotropic Drugs

carries its own risks. Research confirms another common practice of combining a major tranquilliser (neuroleptic) with an antidepressant drug (Michel and Kolakowska, 1981; Edwards and Kumar, 1984). Neuroleptics, however, enhance the side effects associated with antidepressants, e.g. sudden falls in blood pressure. Moreover, they do not have an antidepressant action. In fact, like some of the antihypertensive drugs which they resemble chemically, they can have the reverse action of inducing depression, especially in those prone to this condition. Sleeplessness, anxiety and agitation, common features of a depressive illness, can all be controlled by a single true antidepressant with a sedative effect (e.g. dothiepin or mianserin, given mainly at night).

Attempts to produce an improvement and remission of depression may be in vain, perhaps because of misdiagnosis or ineffectual drug treatment. Alternatively, as Bergmann reports:

> Medication started may be added to because of persistent symptoms of depression, anxiety and hypochondriasis. Ultimately the patient may become the victim of a desperately escalating polypharmacy and admitted to hospital with phenothiazine-induced Parkinsonism and hypotension, delirium induced by anti-Parkinson drugs, gross constipation and dehydration induced by antidepressives, or unsteadiness and ataxia from benzodiazepines with only a few depressive symptoms remaining of the original illness (Bergmann, 1982, p.171).

There are at least 36 antidepressant drugs on the market. Convincing evidence that one antidepressant is superior to others is not available. Many are combination drugs where the dose of the antidepressant is not of adequate potency to reverse a depressive illness. The first antidepressant drug to have a major impact was imipramine (Tofranil) introduced in the late 1950s. It is easily the cheapest antidepressant on the market. Since imipramine, there has been a desperate search for antidepressant drugs with greater efficacy and fewer side effects. Years later, after innumerable trials, none have been found to have a consistent advantage in efficacy over imipramine (Imlah, 1981) or in speed of action. Some, however, have fewer side effects and may be better tolerated by older people.

Newer and more expensive antidepressants, such as trazadone and mianserin, have been particularly recommended for older people, especially in the commercial literature. New, however, does not necessarily mean better, and all these drugs have side effects. The magnitude of these is in part proportionate to the length of time the drug has been on the market.

62

Lithium salts are now used in selected patients with intractable depression. However, in the case of lithium there is a very narrow line between its therapeutic and toxic dose. Treatment must be preceded by renal function tests and other checks; once started, the patient needs close monitoring with repeated lithium blood levels. The addition of other drugs especially diuretics, radically reduces lithium elimination by the kidneys, easily precipitating a severe toxic state. If a diuretic has to be prescribed the lithium should be stopped. Finally, it must always be remembered that the drug easily accumulates when renal function declines.

As with the young, the commonest agent of suicide in the elderly is drug overdose. Tricyclic antidepressants can be lethal in overdosage. This highlights the danger of excessive prescribing in patients with depression. Self-poisoning has been found to be the second most common reason for emergency admission to medical beds (Smith, 1972). Smith estimated in 1972 that over 70,000 cases of self-poisoning may be admitted to hospitals in the United Kingdom each year. The change in the drug used for overdose over the preceding decade was paralleled by the change in national prescribing habits, in particular the increasing use of tranquillisers.

More recently there has been a steep rise in overdosage with antidepresssant drugs, reflecting a massive increase in their prescription (9.5 million prescriptions were issued by general practitioners in England and Wales in 1977). Anxiety is now being expressed that drugs specifically for depressive illnesses are being used indiscriminately (Tyrer, 1978; Prescott and Highley, 1985).

The Complaint of Sleeplessness and the Use of Hypnotics in the Elderly

About 45 per cent of elderly people living at home claim they sleep badly. About 28 per cent of them, mainly women, regularly receive hypnotics. It can help these patients if they know that, though most adults take about 10 minutes to drop off to sleep, by the time they reach 70 it is nearer 20-25 minutes. Old people also have more phases of light sleep (when they may wake up) in comparison with younger people.

In a study in the US, Karacan and Williams (1983) reported that insomnia-related problems were complained of by 50 per cent of persons over the age of 60, compared with 26 per cent of persons 20-29. With 22 million Americans over 65 years, a sizeable number of people are having trouble sleeping; in fact, a mouth-watering number in terms of the market for hypnotics. More older men than older women exhibit the objective changes in EEG (electro-encephalogram) recordings that correspond to poor sleep, yet proportionately twice as many elderly women than men have subjective complaints about sleep. Many elderly people who sleep in the daytime complain of night-time insomnia, instead of daytime hypersomnia. Older persons frequently do not maintain a strict schedule of sleeping at night and staying awake during the daytime.

The clinical importance of sleep disturbance remains largely unknown. The extensive and routine prescribing of hypnotic drugs must be viewed against this background. Many patients will 'select' a physical complaint or 'insomnia' as a 'ticket' to present to their doctor. Prescriptions are still given for the symptom of insomnia alone, without adequate prior history-taking to determine whether the symptom simply reflects poor sleeping habits, physical causes or a psychiatric disorder. Much depends on the doctor's experience and training but even more on the factor of time. Oswald (1984a) recommends that in a doctor's first assessment of the symptom of insomnia, an adequate history may mean being prepared to give 30-60 minutes to find out what has been going on in the patient's life. In contrast, the giving of a prescription can be a very quick transaction. While benzodiazepine hypnotics are relatively safe and effective, stopping them after a short time (Power et al., 1985, found as little as six weeks), and certainly if taken for months, can lead to rebound sleeplessness and daytime anxiety so that the patient mistakenly believes that her initial problem has returned and so presses for further medication.

Prescription policies for hypnotics vary within and between institutions. Oswald, for example, found that the nightly hypnotic intake amongst healthy residents of Edinburgh old people's homes varies from 15 per cent in one home to 50 per cent in another. In a home for the elderly mentally infirm in Birmingham and a psychiatric hospital facility in Galway with a high proportion of elderly patients, no night sedatives as such are prescribed at all. Christopher et al. (1978) found as many as 70 per cent of older people in hospital care in Dundee were on hypnotics.

In a survey of the use of hypnotic drugs in 23 old people's homes in Scotland, one-third of residents had been given hypnotics (mainly nitrazepam) on the night of the survey and almost one half of these were also taking other centrally acting drugs (Morgan and Gilleard, 1981). There was a huge variation - from 10 to 60 per cent - in the 23 different homes in the use of hypnotics. Morgan went on to report that residents who were incontinent, confused or mentally handicapped were less likely to be given hypnotic drugs. It was the least impaired and most active who received most of these drugs. Some staff had obviously discovered that incontinence at night can be induced or exacerbated by night sedation.

There is a tendency to develop tolerance within 3 to 14

days of continuous use of sedative drugs (British National Formulary (BNF), no.3, 1982, p.107). Patients on long term night sedation may have as great or greater difficulty in falling asleep as patients complaining of insomnia, acting as controls, who are on no medication (Kales et al., 1974).

An increased sensitivity to nitrazepam (Mogadon) in old age has been demonstrated by Castleden et al. (1977), and a much altered pattern of drug handling of diazepam (Valium) in old age by Swift et al. (1980) (see Chapter 2). Castleden studied the effect of a single 10 mg oral dose of nitrazepam and compared it with those of a placebo in healthy young adults and old people. The elderly were over 60 with a mean age of 74.7 years. Both the young and the elderly slept better on three successive nights after nitrazepam, but they felt less awake at 12 and 36 hours later. Elderly people made significantly more mistakes in a psychomotor test than did the young, despite similar plasma concentrations of nitrazepam.

However, the particular side effects (in both groups) of mainly sleepiness in the day, unsteadiness/dizziness and nausea were found to be directly correlated with the plasma nitrazepam concentration. When the medication is given more continuously as is the common practice, the more common delay in elimination of the drug in the elderly (leading to accumulation and high plasma and steady state levels) accounts for the clinical finding of a much higher rate of these types of side effects.

The Boston Collaborative Drug Surveillance Program has also demonstrated that the frequency of unwanted depression of the central nervous system following nitrazepam and flurazepam (probably the two commonest night sedatives used in the USA) increased significantly above the age of 70. These unwanted effects in the elderly have also been illustrated by Greenblatt et al. (1977).

One of the main difficulties with the elderly is the risk of drug accumulation, especially with hypnotics that have a long half-life, i.e. those that are, even in normal circumstances, only slowly excreted from the body. Morgan (1982) and Cook et al. (1983) have conducted detailed studies that illustrate the problem. Cook found that, in elderly patients, plasma nitrazepam more than doubled after seven nights of medication compared with that after one night; temazepam went up by 50 per cent in the same period. Both for nitrazepam and temazepam the reaction time was unchanged on the morning after the first dose, but was significantly prolonged after the seventh dose of both hypnotics. The plasma accumulation of the drug was associated with a deterioration in daytime performance.

No doubt the increased sensitivity amongst the elderly, together with higher steady state and plasma levels on continuous treatment, played their part.

A critical view of the use of nitrazepam was made by

Evans and Jarvis back in 1972. They argued, in a letter to the British Medical Journal, that:

Despite statements to the contrary made in advertising literature, nitrazepam (Mogadon) seems a particularly unsuitable hypnotic for old people. [We] have come to recognise a characteristic syndrome of disability caused by nitrazepam, of which the following case is typical.
A 75-year-old lady had been resident in an old people's home for six years. Before admission there she had made a good recovery from a slight left hemiparesis [stroke] and had mild heart failure, well controlled by digoxin, but she was generally ambulant, continent and orientated. She was referred to us with a diagnosis of having suffered a further stroke after two weeks of general mental deterioration, inability to walk and incontinence of urine and faeces. She had become dysarthric [poor speech], confused and disorientated and, if left undisturbed, would sit staring blankly into space. She tended to fall to the left and to stumble when attempting to walk. Specific questioning elicited the information that she looked better and seemed mentally more alert when in bed than when sitting out and that she had been taking one (5 mg) tablet of nitrazepam nightly for at least a year. We advised stopping the nitrazepam and on review three days later she was said to be 'completely her old self' and had gone out on a charabanc trip. After four months she remains well.

The authors went on to say that symptoms suggestive of postural hypotension, i.e. sudden falls in blood pressure on standing, were not uncommon in the elderly on nitrazepam, especially those who already had vascular disease. These changes and their associated symptoms were often unrecognised, patients seldom mentioning to their doctor that they were taking sleeping tablets. Recovery was rapid once the drug was stopped. They thought that nitrazepam was popular because of its rapid effect and that it was widely used in residential homes and elsewhere when it was convenient or necessary for old people to be 'switched off' with the lights. If a department of geriatric medicine sees only the most severe cases of any disease, Evans wondered how many old people in the community were suffering from milder degrees of chronic impairment due to their sleeping tablets. Nitrazepam (Mogadon) is the most commonly used hypnotic in the UK for all age groups. In fact Swift (1982) found that 89 per cent of nitrazepam prescriptions were accounted for by those aged 65 and over. The drug is thus in common use with older people, despite the fact that according to one researcher: 'Nitrazepam has been shown again and again to cause impairment of mental functions, especially in the elderly' (Oswald, 1984a, p.1536).

Conclusion: Long Term use of Psychotropic Drugs and the Problem of Drug Dependency

Williams (1983a), in a survey of patterns of psychotropic drug use, confirmed the increasing population of long-term psychotropic consumers especially among the elderly. Yet Cartwright's two studies of general practice in 1964 and 1977 (Cartwright, 1967; Cartwright and Anderson, 1981) showed that patients were more likely to question whether the doctor was right than they had been 10 years before. She found a significant increase in the proportion of patients who were critical of their doctors for being too inclined to give prescriptions for psychotropic drugs. This reluctance to take such drugs was not so evident among older people.

Drury (1982) reviewed evidence from a variety of sources and came to the conclusion that over the past 10-15 years there had been a marked increase in the proportion of prescriptions that were issued on an 'unseen repeat' basis. This was for all types of drugs but was especially the case with psychotropic drugs. The proportion of psychotropic drug consumers who were receiving prescriptions on a long-term repeat basis increased dramatically from about 30 per cent in 1967/68 to about 60 per cent in 1977/78. Marks (1984) reported that 50 per cent of long-term users of benzodiazepine drugs had not seen their doctor within the previous four months.

It is now being realised that patients can become psychologically and physically dependent on benzodiazepines (Peturrson and Lader, 1981; Tyrer, 1984b), that this number is rising and that it is related to the duration of drug treatment. In turn the duration of treatment has been found to be age- and sex-related (Parish, 1971; Williams, 1983a).

Despite the fact that the efficacy of hypnotics such as the benzodiazepines may decline after 3-12 days (BNF, no.3, 1982, p.107), and that treatment with the benzodiazepines should be short term (Committee for Review of Medicines, 1980), very little change in the number of prescriptions and none in the duration of supply has yet become apparent. Following scares concerning the value of diazepam (Valium) after reports of spontaneous outbursts of violent agression (British Medical Journal leader, 1975), increasing anxiety (Parrott and Kentridge, 1982), and other problems such as insomnia (Kales et al., 1983), restlessness, depression and suicidal ideation (Hall and Joffe, 1972), there has been a 20 per cent fall in diazepam prescriptions. Yet this fall has usually been made up by one or other of the 19 other newer benzodiazepines rushed onto the UK market by the pharmaceutical companies. Some of these 20 drugs are marketed by different companies giving 32 trade preparations for the UK prescriber to choose from in 1984.

In a survey among six GPs, Williams (1983a) studied the duration of drug treatment with psychotropic drugs generally and tranquillisers in particular, this either for the first time ever or for new episodes of disorder. He found that, in the main, treatment with psychotropic drugs was a short-term affair. A survival distribution curve showed that about half the patients had ceased treatment by the end of the first month. Subsequently, however, the rate at which treatment was stopped decreases sharply so that by the end of the follow-up period of six months, about one-fifth of the patients were found to have received drug treatment continuously. The presence of physical illness was not related to the duration of treatment, but older recipients of tranquillisers were likely to receive treatment for a longer period than younger recipients. There was no relationship between the patient requesting drug treatment and duration. He confirmed the marked differences between doctors in their prescribing habits, reiterating that there still was no universal agreement, let alone clear criteria, to enable a doctor to distinguish between 'necessary' and 'unnecessary' psychotropic drug treatment. The suggestion arises that some doctors interact with their patients in such a way as to encourage long-term use. Not all doctors are, it seems, prepared, or even able, to discuss with patients the medicines they prescribe, or possible alternatives to drugs. This situation is worsened with the elderly patient by problems of communication and by altered attitudes of doctors towards the elderly (see Chapters 3 and 4).

Chapter 6

DRUGS FOR HYPERTENSION IN OLDER PEOPLE

Introduction

What is hypertension and what is its meaning for the old and
very old? Blood pressure refers to the pressure at which
blood is pumped from the heart into the main arteries to be
distributed around the body. The blood pressure recording
consists of two readings. The upper reading is the pressure
at the point when the contractions (systole) of the heart
forces the pulse wave of blood through the artery from which
the pressure is recorded. This is known as the systolic
blood pressure. The second reading is the pressure recorded
between the pulse waves when the heart is relaxed, and filled
with blood (diastole) ready for the next pumping action - this
is called diastolic blood pressure. The readings are recorded
as the systolic over the diastolic pressures, e.g. 140/80.
    In the industrialised western world, blood pressure rises
with age, beginning at about 40 years to a peak around the
age of 75. For example, in a British survey the mean blood
pressure at age 75 was found to be 180/95 mm Hg in women
and 165/90 in men, compared with 130/80 in men and women
at age 40 (Hamilton et al., 1954). With an increase in blood
pressure in middle age there is also an increased risk of
problems such as strokes, and heart and kidney failure.
Thus high blood pressure in middle age is a common silent
precursor of ill health and death. Among those over 60,
although this trend tends to continue (as judged by the
Framingham Studies in the USA - Kannel et al., 1976; Kannel
and Gordon, 1978), it is less clear-cut. In those over 70 it
is particularly uncertain. In this chapter we are
concentrating on mild 'essential' or uncomplicated
hypertension, the category where excessive drug treatment is
most likely to occur.
    In addition to uncertainty over just what values of
systolic and diastolic pressure do constitute hypertension in
individuals over 65 (Brocklehurst, 1978), there is current
concern that blood pressure readings vary according to who

69

is doing the measuring (O'Malley, 1985). For example, many patients diagnosed as having mild hypertension at the clinic have normal blood pressure recorded by home measurements (O'Brien et al., 1985; see also Manek et al., 1984). Doctors, in other words, by their very presence, increase the blood pressure when they record it themselves, especially in initial measurements. O'Brien's team concluded that home self-recorded measurements could provide more accurate identification of those patients with borderline raised pressure, i.e. those who do not need antihypertensive drug treatment.

Blood pressure varies a great deal, even for the same individual, with such events as anxiety, exercise, standing, sitting and lying down, as well as a full bladder, pain, cold and drugs unconnected with the control of blood pressure. This variation is even greater among older people.

For the drug industry, hypertension represents an ideal case for mass medication, because it is difficult to make the decision about the cut-off point as regards treatment. As the medical controversy continues, physicians are under considerable pressure to intervene, especially from the drug companies, who interpret the research findings in such a way as to promote prescribing. However, from the age of 70 years different principles apply to the natural history and management of hypertension and the value of treating uncomplicated hypertension is doubtful. From between the ages of 60 and 70, treatment is problematic because of the lack of clear research data. Before the age of 60, however, treatment for severe hypertension would appear to have greater long-term benefit and value to the individual patient.

Although these views appear to represent the norm on the need for treatment or otherwise with older people, as many as half of all people receiving antihypertensive drugs are 65 years or over (Hart, 1982).

In young and middle-aged women there appears no significant benefit from treatment of mild and moderate hypertension (Breckenridge, 1985). Women in this age group should not be given drug treatment pending any new research findings. More beneficial for many hypertensive women would be to relieve the pressures they experience as paid workers and unpaid carers. Such pressures contribute to the problem of smoking amongst women (Sadgrove, 1985), an important contributory agent in hypertension. To illustrate the controversy over the significance of raised blood pressure among older people, a British study (Evans et al., 1980) of 2793 randomly sampled men and women of 65 and over failed to show any significant correlation between arterial pressure and strokes in a two year follow-up. Exclusion of those taking antihypertensives did not affect this result, but previous hypertension in middle life did predict a higher risk of stroke. There are other determinants of stroke which might be noted. For example, there is an unexplained threefold excess of strokes in unskilled compared with professional workers, with parallel north/south geographical differences (Hart, 1979).

There is evidence that in apparently healthy people aged 70-89 neither systolic nor diastolic pressure have any predictive value for survival (Anderson and Cowan, 1976); this includes deaths from cardiovascular or cerebrovascular causes. It seems people found to have high blood pressure but to be otherwise healthy and who have survived 70 years should not automatically receive drug treatment. In fact Williamson (1978) argues that the indications for lowering blood pressure in the over-70s are few and that it must be realised that systolic pressure over 215 mm Hg and diastolic up to 115 mm Hg are not in themselves an indication for treatment.

There is, as observed earlier, a stronger case for treating middle-aged men than middle-aged women. The aim of pressure control is to curtail and prevent heart failure, strokes and renal failure. There is an argument, especially applicable to older people, that a marked <u>fall</u> in blood pressure due to over-energetic or unnecessary treatment can reduce blood flow through vital organs which in turn can have dangerous consequences including further strokes (Jackson <u>et al.</u>, 1976; Jarvis, 1981).

Evidence exists to suggest insufficient caution is in fact taken as regards treatment for hypertension. In one treatment survey, one-third of patients were found to have commenced treatment after just a <u>single measurement</u> (Parkin et al., 1979). In another survey, repeated measurements showed that more than half those believed to be hypertensive in fact had a fluctuating blood pressure called labile or borderline hypertension (Carey <u>et al.</u>, 1976).

Hasty and too few initial measurements could lead to the individual taking unnecessary drugs, which are prone to unpleasant adverse effects, for his or her remaining lifetime. There is therefore a real need for <u>at least three</u> separate blood pressure readings before the diagnosis of hypertension is made. A single reading leads to a misleadingly high prevalence of hypertension (Hart, 1970). It has also been established that patients found initially to have high blood pressure tend with time to remit to pressures more in the normal range (Medical Research Council, 1977).

Who Benefits from Treatment of Hypertension Among the Elderly?

Antihypertensive drugs are, as we have seen, regularly prescribed for older people. Unfortunately, few of the drugs in common use have had any specific geriatric evaluation and there are still no completed randomised controlled trials of treatment in the full age span of the elderly. In fact, we are somewhat ignorant of the pharmacokinetics (drug handling) and pharmacodynamics (drug response) of antihypertensive drugs in this age group (O'Malley and O'Brien, 1980). Barritt has argued that the benefit of medication for the more severe degrees of hypertension is not disputed. Concerning the need for medication in mild hypertension he comments: 'Adjustment for age defies any precision but clearly sustained levels of the order of 160/100 imply a greater risk to longevity and continued health at the age of 40 than at the age of 65' (Barritt, 1982, p.114). He further pointed out that other factors besides drug treatment may be equally important: 'These include male sex, family history, cigarette smoking, social class, diet, lipid levels (fat levels in the blood) and perhaps psychological factors.' He commended a suitable period of observation in years rather than days without treatment (for mild hypertension), adding 'As physicians, we should be as ready to prescribe cessation of cigarette smoking, good sense about diet (including its salt content) and well-judged physical exercise, as to prescribe beta-blockade. We also have to judge occupational stress' (Barritt, 1982, p.114).

The presence of obesity, or the continuation of cigarette smoking, impairs the efficiency of drug treatment, even cancelling out the effect of drugs altogether (MacMahon et al., 1985; Medical Research Council, 1985).

Mild hypertension is always symptomless (Barritt, 1982). Vague symptoms like headache and dizziness are not related to pressure levels; they will not be influenced by lowering the blood pressure and are more likely to respond to reassurance. Again, there is no good evidence that hypotensive therapy prolongs life or reduces the chances of recurrence in patients over 65 who have had a stroke and this should not therefore constitute an indication by itself. Lowering blood pressure in such patients often leads to further deterioration in intellectual capacity (Brocklehurst, 1978).

Evidence For and Against Treatment

The conclusions of the few existing reliable studies have produced conflicting findings. Trials are both difficult to design and carry out. For example, numbers of patients have to be sufficient to allow for statistically significant conclusions to be drawn; in particular, for such subdivisions of patients as those aged 60-70, those 70-80 and those over 80 years.

One such trial was carried out by Sprakling et al. (1981). They studied 540 elderly residents of local authority homes where those with a diastolic pressures of 100 mm Hg or more were randomised to be observed or to be treated with methyldopa. Life table analysis showed that, despite a reduction in mean arterial pressure in the treated group of about 20 mm Hg systolic and 10 mm Hg diastolic, there was no significant difference in outcome between them and the observed (untreated) patients. Indeed the observed group fared somewhat better at all times until the study ended after 90 months. Even residents whose blood pressure had been below 100 mm Hg did no better than the observed hypertensives. In the over-80 age group of the study, those in the highest blood pressure range were associated with a better prognosis.

The study reported by Amery et al. (1985) provides some of the best evidence so far on the initial decision of whether to treat elderly hypertensive individuals. This trial, carried out in 10 European countries, involved 840 patients over the age of 60 years and was conducted by the European Working Party on High Blood Pressure in the Elderly. Entry into the trial, which started in 1972, required the criteria of a sustained systolic blood pressure (averaged over three consecutive occasions) equal to or greater than 160 mm Hg plus a sustained diastolic pressure equal to or greater than 90 mm Hg.

The trial was double-blind (neither the investigator nor the patient knew the nature of the treatment) and the active starting treatment was a combination capsule of a thiazide diuretic with a potassium-retaining diuretic (25 mg hydrochlorothiazide plus 50 mg triamterene) or matching placebo. If the sitting diastolic pressure remained over 90 mm Hg, both active capsule and matching placebo were increased to 2 capsules a day and if necessary up to 4 methyldopa (500 mg) tablets (or matching placebo) could be added.

The results were reviewed every year and only by 1984 had they (in terms of a reduction in heart attacks, strokes and death) reached statistical significance. Basically, although the total mortality rate between the two groups was not significantly different, there was a significant reduction in cardiovascular mortality rate in the treated group. This was due to a significant reduction of cardiac mortality combined with a non-significant reduction in strokes. Put another way, 14 fewer cardiovascular deaths occurred per 1000 patient years in the treated than in the placebo group.

Some questions have been answered by this well conducted trial but others remain unanswered. The European Working Party have yet to break down their figures to assess benefits in narrower age brackets. Many must have been in the 60-70 age range, with the mean age of the 840 patients being 72 years. There were few patients over 80 years. Thus contained within the study are the younger 60-70 year olds and the very old, as well as those with mild raised blood pressure and those with a more extreme form of hypertension.

The important criterion here was that the hypertension was based on both raised systolic and raised diastolic pressure. Many currently treated elderly hypertensives have a raised systolic but not diastolic pressure. Correctly in this trial the systolic pressure was recorded in the erect seated position. Standing would be even better as many older people have a fall on attaining an erect posture (postural hypotension) which if extreme can present them with a very real problem. Even seated a sustained diastolic pressure of over 90 mm Hg in the very elderly is not at all common. The results also only apply to the particular and somewhat unusual treatment regime used in the trial. The relative merits of different classes of antihypertensive agents have not been systematically examined.

A further very large scale trial on the long-term treatment of mild hypertension in 17,354 men and women aged 35-64 years was published in 1985 by the Medical Research Council (MRC)(1985). Several findings in this trial are likely to have a bearing on the issue of treating older people with mild hypertension. Patients were selected whose diastolic blood pressure was in the range 90-109 mm Hg. In brief, the included patient was either treated with a thiazide diuretic (bendrofluazide) or a beta-blocker (propranolol) or a placebo. There were some variations in the two treatment groups to secure a fall of diastolic pressure to below 90 mm Hg. The study was carried out in general practice over five and a half years. The hypertension clinics were well organised and run by nurses. They were successful in tracing defaulters and achieving high compliance levels.

Essentially, active treatment reduced the number of strokes but did not influence the rate of coronary events (contrasting with the European Working Party Trial). Active treatment did not reduce the overall death rate (the death rate for men decreased but that for women increased). Propranolol was more effective in lowering blood pressure in younger than older patients. Smokers taking propranolol showed no reduction in strokes or coronary events. The differences, as pointed out by Breckenridge (1985), in the rate of strokes and coronary events between non-smokers and smokers was impressive, these being much greater than the effects of treatment! In other words stopping smoking may be a more important therapeutic manoeuvre than the prescription of blood pressure lowering drugs.

Because of these differences in the outcome of treatment, Breckenridge (1985) concludes that to treat all women with mild hypertension is not worthwhile. The trial also confirmed (as noted in the section on thiazide diuretics) that the hypotensive effect of thiazides does not appear to be dose-related, although their adverse effects are. As a result, much smaller doses of the drug were recommended. The trial confirmed the high incidence of adverse effects, especially lethargy and impotence in both treatment groups, compared with those taking placebo. Thus the results of this massive and well-conducted trial fell short of a clear-cut answer, suggesting some benefit for stroke reduction but none for coronary events. On this latter point the results were described by Professor Rose, Head of Epidemiology at the London School of Hygiene and Tropical Medicine, as 'disappointing', and he added that 'The main items on our balance sheet would be one stroke per 850 patients per year prevented balanced against troublesome side-effects for one in 20 patients treated for five years' (cited in Pulse, 20 July, 1985, p.8).

From these and other findings, with the use of good clinical judgement there does seem to be potential benefit for some elderly hypertensives whose treatment is initiated over the age of 60 (particularly 60-70) years. This is provided, amongst other things, that their long-term treatment is well monitored, that there is good treatment compliance and that the treatment is not dogged by adverse effects. In the real world, long-term treatment is often not so well monitored (Haines, 1985) and one can only question whether the results would show the same benefit as that shown in the trial of the European Working Party.

To the question as to whether antihypertensives are more likely to do good than harm in the elderly, even in the right circumstances and with proper control, Mitchell has pointed out that it is not known at what age it ceases to be beneficial to treat hypertension, or indeed what is an acceptable blood pressure for old people. He notes:

> The doctor lies who tells a 70 year old man that he knows that his blood pressure needs treating; if he says the same thing to a 70 year old woman, he lies twice over, for the truth is that he can only speak from the most enormous ignorance, as the majority of research on which his advice is based has been done on men and women under 60 (The Times, 30 December 1983).

The Unwanted Effects of Drug Treatment on the Elderly

Side effects from drugs used to treat hypertension in older people (including diuretics) are particularly common. Excessive falls of blood pressure (hypotension) and of blood salts (especially potassium and sodium), as well as dehydration from excessive fluid loss, can lead to incontinence, weakness, immobility, confusion and bed sores. These side effects occur most frequently in older patients (British Medical Journal leader, 1978a; Amery et al., 1978; Beeley, 1980; Lewis, 1984) and may cause considerable distress (Hall, 1973). Any elderly person taking diuretics or hypotensive agents must be examined regularly to avoid

75

overtreatment. For example, potassium levels should be checked, especially if the patient is on a poor diet, shows signs of increasing weakness, or if on digoxin as well as diuretics.

Attacks of dizziness and fainting due to sudden falls of blood pressure on standing are a frequent consequence of the drug treatment. Dizziness is not a symptom of hypertension, but it occurs commonly in older people following a sudden fall of blood pressure on standing or sitting up quickly (postural hypotension).

All antihypertensive drugs can cause postural hypotension in elderly patients. When cerebral arterial pressure falls, as on standing up, an autoregulatory reflex dilates the small arteries in the brain to ensure continued blood flow at a constant rate. When this fails, the subject faints. In the elderly, this autoregulatory function is often deficient and is probably a common cause of postural hypotension, causing giddiness, faintness and confusional states (Wollner et al., 1979). The autoregulatory reflex is shifted upwards in hypertension, which means that high blood pressure should initially be reduced only slowly (if at all) in the elderly. Furthermore, it is wise to measure standing as well as seated pressures during the induction of treatment. The results of this common phenomenon in older people can vary from mild dizziness to a completely disabling condition where the patient becomes bedfast. It is a common cause of falls, especially on rising from a chair or getting out of bed, for example, to go to the toilet.

Elastic stockings might be a far better answer than drugs for dizziness on standing, as well as teaching the patient to get out of bed or chair slowly. In a study by Bradshaw and Edwards (1984) at the Geriatric Department of the Welsh National School of Medicine, some 40 per cent of 71 elderly patients studied showed a significant postural hypotension (most previously unrecognised). Nine patients had a blood pressure on standing of below 100/60. The number of patients with chest infections in the postural hypotension group compared with those without a postural drop was significantly increased.

Acute hypotensive episodes from whatever cause are a common precursor to fatal strokes (Mitchinson, 1980). Over medication with antihypertensive drugs is such a possible cause. Whilst it is generally recognised that the more powerful antihypertensive drugs such as the adrenergic neurone blockers (e.g. guanethidine) and vasodilators (e.g. hydrallazine) are obvious causes of hypotensive episodes, it is often forgotten that postural hypotension occurs frequently in elderly patients treated with beta-blockers as well as the ubiquitous diuretics, particularly in the presence of potassium depletion.

Treating Hypertension

Diuretics
Williamson (1978) has estimated that over one-third of the
elderly population are receiving regular diuretic therapy
('water tablets'). Much of this treatment must be considered
unnecessary. In 54 long-stay in-patients in Cardiff, the
diuretic was stopped; only eight needed to go back on them
(British Medical Journal leader, 1978a). The thiazide
diuretics are the most commonly used. Some unanswered
questions remain as to exactly how they reduce blood
pressure. They promote water loss and decrease blood
volume, thus reducing external cardiac work and arterial
pressure. With a flat dose response curve, more than 1-2
tablets have no further effect on reducing the blood
pressure. In roughly one-quarter of patients they produce a
substantial fall in blood pressure. They increase the action
of all other antihypertensives.

Should they be given in overdose, even marginal
overdose as so easily occurs with older people, no further
reduction of blood pressure is achieved, although their
adverse effects steadily increase. These effects include
excessive loss of sodium and potassium, impaired handling of
glucose, and a rise of blood urates and uric acid (British
Medical Journal leader, 1979a). In consequence, they could
precipitate renal failure or gout (by raising serum urates)
and diabetes (by altering carbohydrate glucose metabolism).
There may be as much as a five-fold increase in diabetes from
diuretics (Caird, 1977b). Impairment of glucose tolerance
occurs more quickly and more universally in older people; 20
per cent of elderly patients show impaired carbohydrate
metabolism. Diuretic use can therefore precipitate mild
diabetes and lead to the addition of oral anti-diabetic agents.
These drugs (such as chlorpropamide) in the elderly have a
long half-life, accumulate and commonly produce confusion and
apparent intellectual failure.

Patients must be warned that a heavy water loss will
follow after taking a diuretic especially if they are in any way
immobile or incontinent. Should the patient become
demoralised with any degree of incontinence it is unlikely that
they will comply with treatment. To give a frail elderly
person a diuretic at the end of the day is a potentially cruel
and hazardous procedure. Getting up in the night to go to
the toilet, thence developing postural hypotension and falling
over, can result in serious injury. In acute heart failure
alternative drugs for use at night (e.g. morphine) should be
sought. According to Hart (1980) diuretics probably increase
the risk of venous thrombo-embolism in old people, an
important and under-diagnosed cause of morbidity and
mortality.

Diuretic drugs lead to loss of excess fluid through the

kidneys. There can also be an associated excessive loss of sodium (hyponatraemia) and potassium (hypokalaemia) which in turn lead to adverse effects. Older people are more prone to hypokalaemia which is partly explained by poor diet (Macleod et al., 1975). The fall in serum potassium usually occurs early, therefore it should be assessed in the first place before and some two months after starting treatment. Other drugs, including some laxatives, increase the loss of potassium.

The safety margin of low blood potassium is probably reduced in older people (Williams, 1985). In younger adults, a low limit of 3.0 mmol/litre is compatible with health whilst levels in the range 3.0 - 3.5 in the elderly have been shown to be associated with postural hypotension leading to dizziness, fainting and falls (Hamby et al., 1980). They may also suffer from other symptoms due to low potassium levels, which include lethargy, apathy and rapid fatigue, all seriously impairing the quality of life in old age.

Potassium blood levels are less likely to fall with diuretics if the patient has an adequate and varied diet. Meat, vegetables and fruit are good sources of potassium and if they are available and eaten by the older person, potassium supplements are unnecessary. Potassium supplements are poor safeguards and have to be taken at least three times a day. They are unpalatable and patient compliance is amongst the worst of any tablets prescribed for geriatric patients (Macdonald et al., 1977). Even expensive effervescent preparations are not liked. They can lead to toxicity from excess potassium, which may lead to weakness, confusion and disturbance of heart rhythms. Expensive combined diuretic and potassium preparations do not contain enough potassium and should not be used (Beeley, 1980). The amount of diuretic usually present is not sufficient to produce hypokalaemia and the amount of potassium too small to prevent or correct hypokalaemia!

Newer potassium-sparing diuretics (e.g. amiloride and triamterene) are sometimes recommended as they do not influence the total body potassium deficit which occurs in congestive heart failure (Davidson, 1978). Should potassium supplements be added to these drugs there is a real risk of fatal intoxication with potassium (hypokalaemia) (Greenblatt and Kock-Weset, 1973). They usually have to be given in combination with a thiazide diuretic to achieve a sufficient hypotensive effect. The combination preparations are less effective than when given separately and the thiazide dose is also more than one would use initially with older people. However, for those elderly hypertensives in poor general health, the particular combination of thiazide and triamterene was favourably reported on in preventing hypokalaemia by the European Working Party on Hypertension in the Elderly (Amery et al., 1978). Those combination drugs widely prescribed in the UK are: amiloride and hydrochlorothiazide as 'Moduretic' and triamterene and hydrochlorothiazide as 'Dyazide'.

There is continuing controversy over which diuretic is most suitable for use with older people. The combination drugs, for example, are very expensive. Moreover, it has to be remembered that the very small dose of a thiazide (only) diuretic in an otherwise healthy elderly patient does not usually cause potassium depletion. Comparative published studies do not exist to guide the practitioner. With the thiazide diuretic alone an acceptable dietary salt restriction reduces the risk of hypokalaemia and further helps the hypotensive effect. Such a modest reduction in salt intake can be achieved by avoiding salty foods and by not adding salt to food at the table (this area is further reviewed in Chapter 10). The fixed-ratio combinations are inflexible and therefore difficult to use effectively.

There are some drug combinations currently advocated containing three different antihypertensive agents in the same tablet. Each of these has a different time course of action and evidence of synergistic or even additive effect has rarely been looked for in these kinds of medication. Despite this, the combined drugs are used in massive amounts in the elderly. Doctors readily remember brand names. For example, Smith Kline and French chose Dyazide for their new diuretic; it is so close to thiazide that it is quickly remembered and readily trusted.

The combined drug Moduretic (amiloride plus hydrochlorothiazide) designed to prevent hypokalaemia has recently been found to produce a significant fall in plasma sodium (hyponatraemia), which can lead to serious problems including apathy, mental confusion and weakness without necessarily being recognised as a drug side effect (Millson et al., 1984). Millson and his colleagues suggest that Moduretic should not be in general use with elderly patients and they favour simply a thiazide with potassium supplement when indicated.

The very potent loop diuretics such as frusemide, which act on a different part of the renal apparatus, cause an excessively large or rapid diuresis which may profoundly reduce cardiac output (Lewis, 1984), causing weakness, confusion and deteriorating renal function. They can also cause deafness in large doses and should be used sparingly in the very elderly. Interestingly, a Junior Health Minister, Geoffrey Finsburg, told Parliament (March 1983) that the NHS could save £30 million a year if just nine top brands of medicines were prescribed by generic name: Lasix, one of the five brands of frusemide (a loop diuretic), the most heavily promoted and most expensive brand, held the first position of these nine top brands of medicines, where the possible total savings alone was given at £6.4 million (Medawar, 1984).

The widely prescribed NSAIDs can blunt the effect of diuretics; this is because these drugs cause salt and water retention (Ramsay, 1984). If an NSAID is added to a diuretic in a patient with severe left heart failure or hypertension, weight gain, worsening oedema or an increase in blood pressure may result. These drugs counteract the response to all antihypertensive drugs.

Diuretics are frequently given to elderly people who have mild ankle oedema totally unrelated to congestive heart failure. Since this is due to immobility and poor venous circulation (e.g. varicose veins), diuretics are inappropriate and unhelpful.

Brown and McGregor (1981) highlighted the problems surrounding the perpetuation and unnecessary use of diuretics when given for oedema (typically shown by swelling of the ankles). Diuretics act on the kidney to cause sodium and water loss. With long-term administration of diuretics, compensatory mechanisms may last several days, whereas the action of the diuretic is much shorter and generally only lasts a few hours. Thus, marked sodium retention occurs on stopping the diuretic, which can be sufficient to cause oedema, convincing the patient and often the doctor that diuretics are essential. This situation is particularly seen in women initially given diuretics for mild ankle swelling or, more commonly, because they are overweight.

Richards (1979) states that 'even with great care it is sometimes difficult to avoid making patients ill with diuretics. The usual cause is failure to reduce the dose of diuretic; normally a diuresis is more difficult to induce than to maintain and it is usually both possible and desirable to reduce the dosage during treatment. Diuretic treatment should always be reviewed periodically to ensure that the dose is appropriate and indeed that the treatment is still necessary at all' (Richards, 1979, p.1128). This is particularly true when other strongly protein-bound drugs are given that increase the plasma concentration of free diuretic by displacement. As we saw in Chapter 2, the free component of the drug in the plasma is the pharmacologically active component.

Beta-blockers
Despite being widely used, there is evidence that the drugs known as beta-blockers should be prescribed only with caution in the treatment of hypertension in older people. Beta-blockers reduce heart output and should be used reluctantly in the elderly because they induce low output heart failure. They can produce a marked slowing of the heart (bradycardia) which may lead to insufficient blood flow through the brain, leading to fatigue and confusional states. Beta-blockers provide a good example of drugs that can effect other disease states. They can make diabetic control more difficult, increase the likelihood of bronchospasm (asthma) in

patients with chronic bronchitis and exacerbate peripheral vascular disease (Dunn, 1984). Many older people experience cold hands and feet and this can be worsened through impaired circulation caused by beta-blockers. They can also upset the precarious neuromuscular balance of the elderly bladder and may cause incontinence.

It seems that beta-blockers are handled differently in the body of the older person from that of the younger adult. Castleden et al. (1975) showed that after a 40 mg dose of propranolol (a commonly used beta-blocker) peak blood levels were four times higher in the elderly than in the young. Likewise, the half life of elimination in the elderly was substantially longer (see Chapter 2). Though we have little evidence on the newer beta-blocking drugs in this age group, atenolol is better tolerated in the elderly (British Medical Journal leader, 1978b) and it can be given once a day by oral administration. The antihypertensive effect of beta-blockers is antagonised (as with most antihypertensive drugs) by the widely used NSAIDs. Beta-blockers affect the ability of the liver to break down to inactive substances other drugs the patient might be taking. This occurs because the beta blockers themselves can slow down or conversely accelerate the enzyme concerned with the breakdown of those additional drugs. This in turn can decrease or increase the blood concentration of the second drug.

Methyldopa

For resistant hypertension, a number of other drugs can be used in the elderly; however, the higher risks of adverse effects have to be constantly weighed against possible advantage. Methyldopa has a potent antihypertensive effect which results from a central action leading to peripheral vasodilation. It is occasionally given in combination with a diuretic but this particular preparation is incompletely absorbed. Tiredness, a frequent sequela, becomes a real hazard in drivers and old people. Drowsiness is much commoner in elderly patients and this may become severe if the drug is not withdrawn (Caird, 1977b). The drowsiness can be partially overcome by prescribing one evening dose, instead of three times a day and this is just as effective in producing a reduction in blood pressure (Wright et al., 1976). Besides drowsiness, severe depression and other psychiatric disturbances, impaired liver function and postural hypotension are not uncommon. Sexual dysfunction with failure of erection has been reported in nearly half the men taking methyldopa. No class of antihypertensive drug seems free from an effect on sexual function in men and this includes diuretics (British Medical Journal, leader, 1979b). Impotence was found to occur in 43 per cent of men taking methyldopa, compared with 17 per cent in untreated hypertensives and 7 per cent of a healthy male population of comparable age (Melville and Johnson, 1982).

Besides life-threatening falls in blood pressure, many other side effects have been reported with methyldopa, in fact the computer profile includes 100 separate adverse effects divided into ten categories covering almost all bodily systems (Melville and Johnson, 1982). These include serious autoimmune effects (haemolytic anaemia, hepatitis and granulocytopaenia).

According to Medawar (1984) generic prescribing of methyldopa instead of by brand name Aldomet could save the NHS £5.7 million per annum. Aldomet is another in the top nine brands of medicines prescribed that we discussed earlier, yet for the elderly hypertensive, especially those commencing treatment for the first time, it is not recommended and 'hardly ever needed' (Jarvis 1981).

Vasodilator Drugs
There are other second and third line drugs used to treat severe resistant hypertension. Some act by dilating small arteries in the 'tree' of the arterial circulation; this reduces peripheral resistance to the work of the heart and thus the blood pressure. Vasodilator drugs (e.g. hydralazine and prazosin) have been little studied in the elderly, yet found useful in younger patients. Side effects are common; they can be reduced by starting with a low dosage and increasing slowly. An important new group of drugs are the calcium antagonists (e.g. nifedipine) which may have many important effects on the cardiovascular system. Among other effects such as the relief of angina, they are effective in the treatment of hypertension by dilating arterioles (small arteries). Their mode of action is complex and not completely understood in general, let alone in the elderly.

There are many pitfalls for the elderly hypertensive. Treatment results of hypertension in the elderly after stroke are conflicting and can be positively harmful (Carter, 1970; Adams, 1965). Erratic control may increase the risk of organ damage and lead to a further stroke (Beevers et al., 1973). The risk from erratic control might well be higher in older patients and justifies caution in treating patients with poor medication compliance.

Digitalis Preparations
Sir William Withering introduced digitalis into medical practice nearly 200 years ago. The preparations were first derived by a Midlands herbalist from foxglove leaves. Digoxin, the best known of these preparations is widely used, especially among the elderly. It has a dramatic effect in heart failure by increasing the force of contraction of the heart. Although not directly indicated for uncomplicated hypertension, it is used when heart failure develops as a consequence of hypertension. There are of course other indications. To be

effective, digoxin must be in the tissues at a concentration close to that at which toxic effects occur. That is, there is a narrow therapeutic range (or index) and side effects are very common. Toxic effects occur particularly in the elderly. Dall (1970) recorded their presence in 27 out of 80 elderly patients being treated with a maintenance dose of digoxin. The problem is complicated because the elderly not uncommonly experience toxic effects when the blood level is in the therapeutic range; this is presumably due to an intrinsic increase in tissue sensitivity (Lancet leader, 1983).

The use of digoxin in the elderly has been hotly debated over recent years, especially as the mainstay of the treatment of congestive heart failure. Five per cent of the elderly are taking digoxin and toxicity is common, both at home and in hospital. Symptoms of digoxin poisoning can be very different in the elderly compared with younger age groups (Dall, 1965). Apathy, weakness, confusion and other psychological disturbances are more common than the classical symptoms of nausea, vomiting and slowing of the heartbeat (Toghill et al.,1974).

Hurwitz and Wade (1969) have reported on the very high incidence of adverse reactions to digitalis preparations. In their hospital study, 20 per cent of patients had adverse reactions, the elderly and women compared with men had most reactions. The risk rate was greater in patients who were also given diuretics, a finding in accord with the known pharmacology of these drugs.

Hurwitz (1969b) also found that digitalis preparations were one of the commonest causes of admission to hospital for adverse drug reaction in middle aged and elderly people. These were described as the inevitable consequence of the therapeutic efficacy of the drug, which the patient seldom recognised to be a result of drug therapy. She went on to say that 'the size of this problem has not been fully appreciated' (Hurwitz, 1969b, p.540).

The Glasgow Drug Surveillance Programme again found that some 20 per cent of patients receiving digoxin developed toxicity, the majority being over 65. In one study of 42 elderly patients, only one third of them were found to be receiving an ideal dose (Whiting et al., 1978). Most geriatricians now treat congestive heart failure in sinus rhythm (normal rhythm) with simple diuretic therapy and omit digoxin (Williamson, 1978). Williamson points out that, in the limited number of older patients needing continuous treatment with digoxin, it must be given in smaller doses. This is especially so if renal function is significantly low, for instance when the patient has heart failure as is usually the case when digoxin is prescribed. In any case renal function declines with age (Chapter 2) and lowered measures of renal clearance are more the norm than the exception for older people.

Digoxin stays longer in the body of an elderly person than in a young one. It readily accumulates. Ewy et al. (1969) found that the plasma half-life in men of 73-81 years was 73 hours but only 51 hours in younger subjects. A reduction in kidney filtration rate readily leads to digoxin accumulation and intoxication as excretion falls. This can follow simply from dehydration as well as many other causes, including that of the ageing of the kidney. Even today complete knowledge of the pharmacokinetics (drug handling) of digoxin in the elderly is not available (MacDonald and MacDonald, 1982). Evidence suggests that digoxin is handled differently in the elderly, where there is a declining renal function and an altered volume of distribution of digoxin throughout the body (Caird and Kennedy, 1977).

Whatever the cause, the drug handling becomes very complicated with the ever-present risk of a minimal increase over the therapeutic dose producing in time severe, sometimes lethal, toxic effects. Even when there are advantages of digoxin in the acute phase of a cardiac illness, the indication for long-term use of digoxin (a common practice) is much less obvious in the elderly. Dall (1970) for example found in a group of elderly patients on long-term therapy that almost three quarters showed no harm through stopping it. He went on to say that elderly patients on maintenance digoxin treatment should be reviewed and, in the absence of a known primary cardiac lesion, an attempt should be made to withdraw digoxin.

Graduated programmes of introducing digoxin in the elderly are fraught with difficulty. Programmes of taking the drug several times a day, or alternate days or 'take for 5 days and omit 2', are really unnecessary in the elderly, and frequently lead to incomplete compliance, i.e. the patient moves towards taking the tablets at random intervals. The introduction of smaller dose tablets makes a sensible once-daily dose possible for the elderly.

Digoxin is commonly prescribed to the elderly and there is good evidence that this is often without clinical justification (Landahl et al., 1977; Dunn, 1984). Digoxin treatment requires regular review. A substantial number of older people can have the drug discontinued without any detrimental effects (Dall, 1970; Johnson and McDevitt, 1979). Even when there were good grounds for starting digoxin, the Liverpool Therapeutic Group (1978) showed that if the heart failure had resolved and the heart was in regular rhythm it was still possible to withdraw digoxin safely. Again because digoxin is so toxic in the elderly, peripheral vasodilator drugs have recently been introduced and found safer. Arteriolar vasodilation reduces peripheral vascular resistance, which, for the failing heart, provides scope for improving cardiac function.

Finally, Jarvis concludes that:

Too many old people are given digoxin and many of them are given too much of it. The indications for digoxin are simple: first to control the ventricular rate in patients' atrial fibrillation; and, second (much less commonly needed), to abolish or prevent paroxysmal atrial tachycardia. Digoxin is almost always unnecessary for patients whose hearts are in sinus (normal) rhythm. The correct dose of digoxin is the smallest dose that will maintain a satisfactory heart rate (Jarvis, 1981, p.314).

He points out further that the elderly vary greatly in their response to digoxin and the dose must be tailored to each individual. It is the continuous use of digoxin that particularly poses hazards for the elderly. Digoxin highlights the general motif that chronic care for the elderly is constantly changing care.

Conclusion: Polypharmacy and the Problem of Dependency

Regimes of combined hypotensive therapy in the elderly hold real disadvantages because of their increasing complexity. The appropriate dose of a single drug is better than a combination of drugs. There are also problems with any other drugs that the patient might be taking. As has been said, the multiple pathology of the elderly is a standing temptation to polypharmacy. Antidepressants, phenothiazine neuroleptics (major tranquillisers) and levodopa for Parkinson's disease may all potentiate hypotensive drugs. Problems of falls due to postural hypotension may arise when they are combined; and a dangerous rebound of hypertension can occur when one of these drugs is stopped suddenly. Hypotensive drugs in their turn may affect the elimination of other drugs by reduced renal perfusion. They may for example reduce clearance of drugs with a narrow therapeutic margin, such as digoxin or lithium, and poisoning effects will soon follow due to their accumulation.

The question remains open as to whether treatment of hypertension should be initiated over the age of 65 and is certainly dubious over 70 in the absence of causally related symptoms and organ failure (Hart, 1980). Yet in one study of elderly patients with hypertension, the average number of drug categories used per patient increased consistently with increasing age from 1.6 categories of drugs in patients under 70 to 2.6 categories in patients over 84 (Hale et al., 1979). Caird (1977b) recommends that patients should be carefully reassessed at about 70 years and their blood pressure closely monitored for the effect of reduction or cessation of medication. Psychological dependence may have been instilled by the initial terror of the consequences of increased blood pressure and of not taking their medication regularly at the commencement of treatment years before. All the patient's circumstances must be assessed, especially at the initiation of treatment in the first place, with the motto that at all times one should not do more harm than good.

The rise in the prescription of antihypertensive drugs has outstripped all others except tranquillisers, which themselves are often used in the treatment regime for high blood pressure. From 1966 to 1975, the NHS bill for antihypertensive drugs rose from £6 million to £20 million and reached nearly £63 million in 1984; that for diuretics went from £4 million to £20 million, and then to £56 million over the same time intervals.

A similar escalation of antihypertensive drugs has occurred in other parts of the world, where in many instances amongst the top five drugs prescribed at least four are used in hypotensive treatment (Melville and Johnson, 1982). Melville and Johnson argue that the pharmaceutical industry still considers hypertension to be the most important world-wide area for expansion. In the UK they say that the blood pressure boom has brought drug companies increased sales revenues of about £180 million over a ten-year period. They write further that 'One would expect the bogey of heart disease to be in retreat, if not stopped in its tracks by this explosion of attention and expenditure. Yet in Britain in 1979, deaths from heart disease reached new record levels' (Melville and Johnson, 1982, p.84), and they are probably higher than anywhere else in the world (Catford and Ford, 1984).

Chapter 7

DRUGS FOR SENILE DEMENTIA

Introduction

Dementia is usually an irreversible condition of reduced
cerebral (brain) function resulting from organic damage to the
brain. There is a variety of causes of dementia, but the
commonest by far in older people is senile dementia or
Alzheimer's disease, often called senile dementia of the
Alzheimer type (SDAT). How to respond to the increase in
senile dementia is a significant problem for health and social
services. It is a major issue facing ageing populations
(primarily because it precludes independent life) and it will
continue to increase considerably in the UK during the next
quarter of a century. Dementia has a devastating effect both
on the sufferers and on those members of the patient's family
who have to watch the disintegration of the personality of
someone close to them.

Dementia - How common is it?

It has been estimated that between half and one million people
in the UK suffer from dementia. It is present in 2 per cent
of those 65-70 years, but experienced by 20 per cent of those
over 80 years. The majority of elderly patients suffering
from dementia live in the community. Of those people with
severe dementia of any type, fewer than one in five are cared
for in institutions (Kay et al., 1964). Helgason (1977) found
that although 25 per cent of elderly patients with severe
organic brain syndromes came to the attention of the
psychiatric services in Iceland, only 10 per cent of those with
less than severe syndromes did so.
    The focus of our attention here is on dementia, but we
should not forget that the surveys of its prevalence in the
UK have also made us aware of the high level of mental
function of the majority of older people, with cognitive
(intellectual) processes remaining substantially unimpaired.

Dementia - What is it?

Dementia has been defined as 'an acquired global impairment of intellect, memory and personality but without impairment of consciousness' (Lishman, 1978). It is a slowly progressive condition leading to a range of intellectual, emotional and behavioural changes (Gilleard, 1984). These changes may include difficulty in remembering, speech disturbances, extreme anxiety and agitation, restlessness, and aggression and hostility.

Not suprisingly, with such a range of behaviours, mistakes in diagnosis are quite common - estimated at 10-20 per cent in the 65-75 age range. Conditions mistaken for dementia include drug intoxication states, hypothyroidism, depressive illness, alcholism and a variety of other problems frequently eminently treatable. Careful evaluation of patients labelled as demented has shown that between 2 and 10 per cent are actually depressed (Hier and Caplan, 1980). Extracerebral disease, that is disease outside the brain, which can of course give rise to an organic psychosis or mental illness on its own account, may aggravate symptoms due to senile dementia.

Impaired hearing or eyesight, poor diet, drug intoxication states, depression or apathy associated with social isolation, may all complicate the picture. Their alleviation will undoubtedly be appreciated by the older person and reduce the dependency on others or the immediate demand for institutional care.

Surveys in this country and others have all shown senile dementia of the Alzheimer type (SDAT) to be the most common type of dementia. The next most common type is that once referred to as arteriosclerotic dementia and now called multi-infarct dementia (MID), accounting for about 17 per cent of those dying in institutions (Tomlinson et al., 1970).

Senile Dementia Alzheimer Type

In Alzheimer's disease there is a slow progression in mental disability and capacity for daily living. This is associated with an atrophy, or wastage and shrinkage, of the brain and enlargement of the central spaces or ventricles. The weight of the brain may be reduced by one-fifth or more, accompanied by a massive loss of nerve cells especially in the hippocampal region where memory processes are consolidated. There is a quantitative relationship between the clinical features of senile dementia and the extent of the pathological changes. There are characteristic degenerative changes in the cerebral cortex (the highest part of the brain) that can be viewed with a microscope. The changes in the brain tissues are not localised and involve many kinds of cells. Moreover, the blood vessels themselves show no sign of disease.

The cause of senile dementia and hence the treatment remain unknown (Bowen and Davidson, 1984). Some (but far too little) research is being carried out in this area. The subtleties of senile dementia are considerable and to date there is no agreed sub-classification (Byrne and Arie, 1985). Changes in neurotransmitter (chemical messenger) metabolism, especially of acetylcholine, have been found. There is evidence that acetylcholine is one of the major transmitter substances primarily responsible for higher mental function within the brain. Studies of biopsy tissue have shown that there is a marked reduction of choline acetyl transferase (the enzyme responsible for acetylcholine synthesis) activity which relate to the degree of degenerative changes of the nerve cells and mental function scores of the patients. Attempts to reduce memory impairments in clinical trials by cholinergic stimulation have not been therapeutically successful (Green and Costain, 1981; Bartus et al., 1982; Castleden, 1984). Cholinergic drug treatment to compensate for the known deficit of acetylcholine in senile dementia (SDAT), has been reviewed by Bryne and Arie. They report that: 'Clinical trials of precursors (of acetylcholine) have been almost uniformly negative, and giving such substances causes practical problems as they are bulky - and it is also debatable whether such agents increase the amount of central cholinergic activity' (Byrne and Arie, 1985, p.1846). Research must continue and it may be insufficient to activate only one neurotransmitter at a time when several systems are disturbed.

In dementia there is a decline in cerebral blood flow. Initially, this decline was thought to be the cause of dementia. However, recent work has shown that the decreased flow is secondary to the decreased metabolic demands of cerebral tissue, that is, there is an initial intrinsic reduction in the use of oxygen by the brain tissue that precedes and in fact probably initiates the fall in cerebral blood flow. The theoretical argument that increasing blood flow improves brain function no longer holds true. In fact, no benefit has accrued to patients with the expensive and heavily promoted vasodilator drugs.

Despite the finding of reduced choline activity in the brain, the actual cause and relentless progress of the disease remain an unsolved problem. As yet there is no practical pharmacological means of enhancing cholinergic activity and so improving memory (Smith and Swash, 1982). Dietary supplements of choline or lecithin (a precursor of choline) as a means of enhancing cholinergic activity have not produced beneficial results in experiments conducted for several weeks and there is no convincing evidence that long-term administration of these compounds results in any sustained amelioration of the symptoms of the disease (Swash, 1983).

Multi-infarct Dementia

The term 'cerebral arteriosclerosis', or 'hardening of the arteries of the brain', as applied to mental deterioration in the elderly is misleading and inaccurate (Hachinski et al., 1974). This leads to an image of arteriosclerosis causing a relentless strangulation of the blood supply of the brain as the cause of 'senility'. Blanket treatment with vaso active drugs has ensued from this assumption. When vascular disease is responsible for dementia it is through the occurrence of multiple small or large cerebral infarcts. This blockage of small arteries with the death of brain tissue beyond (an infarct) is invariably due to thrombo-embolism (blood clots) stemming from arteries outside the brain and often in the heart (Hachinski et al., 1974). Actual disease in the small arteries at the base of the brain (arteriosclerosis) is a rare precursor of the manifestation of dementia in old age.

Multi-infarct dementia is a condition that sometimes comes unheralded, but more often follows a steplike fashion after a series of strokes during which specific blood vessels become temporarily or permanently blocked. Initial mental and neurological deficits may with time diminish to a greater or lesser extent. As stated earlier the primary disease is invariably outside the brain. This may be in the heart or sometimes a consequence of long-standing hypertension from middle life (especially in men) characterised by abrupt episodes which lead to weakness, slurred speech, altered gait and other local signs, namely a stroke.

Investigation may allow for more precise diagnosis of the type of dementia and then more accurate prognosis and rational symptomatic treatment. Senile dementia Alzheimer type and multi-infarct dementia, although very different in terms of pathology, can sometimes be extremely difficult to separate in the clinical situation and sometimes occur together.

In reviewing the more recent information gathered from high-technology medical research Byrne and Arie conclude that in multi-infarct dementia: 'such patho-physiological (disease processes) findings call into question the current use of cerebral metabolic enhancers and centrally acting vasodilators. Some centrally acting vasodilators (for example, isoxsuprine) are still being recommended for the treatment of cerebrovascular disorders, but there is neither a scientific rationale nor clinical evidence for such a practice' (Byrne and Arie, 1985, p.1845). Likewise they go on to point out the total lack of agreement over the practical benefits to patients of drugs that enhance cerebral metabolism.

The Treatment Value of Drugs

Before considering treatment it is essential to be sure that the patient does, in fact, have a progressive senile dementia (whether Alzheimer type or multi-infarct dementia). There may be a remedial depressive illness or a drug intoxication state (e.g. from digoxin poisoning) or other intercurrent illness. All these conditions need treating whether or not there is an underlying senile dementia present.

Unfortunately, Tom Arie's statement of 1973 that 'There are no specific drugs for dementia' still holds true (Byrne and Arie, 1985). Drug treatment such as with diuretics, anti-hypertensive drugs, anti-parkinsonian drugs and digoxin can aggravate the effects of senile dementia. Many drugs, whether called 'cerebral vasodilators' or 'cerebral activators', are claimed to arrest intellectual decline and to improve behavioural disturbances associated with the failing brain. The list of drugs on the market is extensive as is the sophisticated chemical rationale on how they might work. Despite laboratory findings that they have an action on the brain chemistry or vasculature, none can be recommended for routine use in patients with brain impairment (Drug and Therapeutics Bulletin, 1975; Byrne and Arie, 1985). The thoughtless prescription of these drugs as placebos is expensive, unnecessary and can lead to unpleasant side effects. What is worse they can lead to a complacent attitude in instituting other more useful remedial measures.

Cerebral or Peripheral Vasodilator Drugs

In 1982, the NHS paid for £2.5 million prescriptions for 'vasodilators and vasoconstrictors' at an average of 10 each. Britain has, in fact, become a profitable market for such drugs. This contrasts with Sweden and Norway where sales are virtually non-existent, although in West Germany these drugs have also achieved record sales (Dukes, 1984). Peripheral vasodilator drugs (PVDs) are meant to improve blood circulation in the brain and the limbs. Besides dementia, they are used to treat a variety of numbing or painful conditions which immobilise and handicap mainly older people. PVDs can improve circulation by dilating healthy blood vessels. Unfortunately, the evidence suggests that they do not work where most needed, when blood vessels either in the brain or in the extremities are diseased. If blood vessels are diseased, PVDs may actually do more harm than good: by improving circulation in healthy blood vessels they may divert blood from diseased to non-diseased areas, the so-called 'steal effect'. Some vasodilators have actually been found to decrease total blood flow to the brain.

PVDs are contraindicated in acute stroke because, as we have seen above, the blood supply may be further diminished to the brain. After strokes, with time the degree of reversibility diminishes and in the chronic stage there is overwhelming doubt about the value of such drugs, despite massive usage. These drugs do not consistently increase cerebral blood flow in doses that can be tolerated by patients. Where they do, and then only transiently (immediately) after taking the drug, usually in high dosage, they do actually increase the total cerebral blood flow but it is highly doubtful if this includes the ischaemic (damaged) area of brain tissue beyond the small artery blockage (George and Hall, 1981).

Despite problems with their use and doubts as to their efficacy, vasodilators are widely promoted for their alleged value with groups such as older people. They are among the most profitable drugs on the world market (Lloyd-Evans et al., 1978). The NHS currently spends around three-quarters of a million pounds per year (mostly for the elderly) on dihydroergotoxine mesylate (Hydergine), one of the brand-leaders in this market. Yet according to one researcher: 'There is no theoretical rationale to support the use of vasodilator drugs in senile dementia' (Hier and Caplan, 1980). The clinical justification has also been questioned (BNF, 1983, no.6, p.90).

Hydergine has been shown in animal research to influence enzymes involved in intermediary stages of metabolism in certain brain cells. In several studies in patients with dementia it has been shown to exert no significant clinical effect despite some alterations detectable on the electroencephalograph (EEG). This drug is not without risk. It is an ergot compound and prolonged use can result in peripheral gangrene, especially if there is pre-existing peripheral vascular disease (Goodman and Gilman, 1980). It can also produce serious falls in blood pressure and slowing of the heart rate.

Events have continued to allow the commercial life of these drugs for the treatment of senile dementia to be extended. Some vasodilator drugs have been found in laboratory conditions to activate various chemical changes not dissimilar to those that occur in brain tissue itself. A new lease of life has been proposed for them by the industry on this basis and without doubt there is worthy theoretical interest in this area. The theory behind these drugs is that by improving the utilisation of glucose and oxygen within the brain cells they will improve the function of the compromised brain. However, research has some way to go before finally demonstrating their value for older people with dementia.

It is salutory to remember that there are other aspects of treatment and management of senile dementia besides drugs. As the Macdonalds note:

It is very important that the prescribing of doubtful drugs does not lull the medical practitioner into a false sense of security, obscuring other more important facets of treatment. Where these patients are being cared for at home they place a great strain on their families. Good social support is essential: holiday relief, washing services if incontinence is a problem, etc. Support groups for families can also be a great boon. It behoves all doctors involved with this problem to deal with it with compassion and to press for adequate provision of essential support services (Macdonald and Macdonald, 1982, p.81).

Other Drugs Including Sedatives and Neuroleptics

Despite the current lack of knowledge it may be important to use limited symptomatic treatment in dementia, first, for those patients who suffer from extreme restlessness or from an altered sleep rhythm (sleeping in the day and up at night); secondly, to manage the associated physical conditions. The drugs of some value here include hypnotics and very small doses of neuroleptics or major tranquillisers (e.g. promazine, or thioridazine). Some argue that sedation should be avoided as much as possible because these drugs often increase confusion by diminishing the patient's alertness.

When using potent neuroleptic drugs one has to strive to obtain that precarious balance before reducing the quality of life of the patient to one of marked drowsiness and inertia, and therefore increasing the work of physical management because the patient has become more immobile, incontinent and in need of heavy nursing care.

Neuroleptics given by mouth or by depot injection, for example every two weeks, produce a high incidence of parkinsonism (see Chapter 5). However, where the behavioural disturbance is considerable (e.g. extreme restlessness and apparent anguish) successful results have been obtained with very small doses of depot injection (Gaspar 1980). In all these patients the drug regime needs to be revised regularly; reductions of medication may ultimately be more effective than additions (Arie, 1973).

Conclusion

Senile dementia has only recently come under intense investigation. Such benefits as have been achieved with drugs in the treatment of dementia and its associated confusion are minimal and of little practical importance, and are usually not sustained (Arie, 1981). At present a specific treatment is not known, yet knowledge about relieving some of the distressing consequences of the conditions is gradually being built up and not all of this is by drugs.

Of the newer agents that have been suggested to overcome the basic biochemical deficit in senile dementia (SDAT) the basis for their use is in most cases tenuous. Byrne and Arie conclude in their review of this area that: 'The current generation of "antidementia drugs" is heterogeneous, containing both drugs of great theoretical interest and of rational derivation and others that seem inherently less likely to be relevant or useful. For the present even those few that have shown some consistent improvements seem to offer neither sufficiently practical nor sufficiently sustained benefits to justify their general use outside a research setting' (Byrne and Arie, 1985, p.1846).

The report of The Royal College of Physicans stated that: 'Research into the best means of symptom control is as important in the short to medium term as fundamental investigation into the causes of senile dementia is in the long term' (Royal College of Physicians, 1981, p.15). Finally, Dukes, in a review of drugs for senile dementia, concluded that: 'We must begin to decide which existing products should have more time to prove themselves and which are just useless.' By 1990, he suggested, 'society should ensure that it either pays less for [such] drugs or gets more benefit in return' (Dukes, 1984).

Chapter 8

CONTROLLING DRUGS:
IMPROVING PROFESSIONAL PRACTICE

Introduction

In this chapter we shall examine alternatives to the present state of prescribing for older people. The alternatives reviewed will include the general philosophy of the prescribing process, the principles underlying better prescribing practices, the prevention of adverse drug reactions, and the monitoring of drug treatment. The need for collaboration to attain these goals, especially between different professional groups, will also be examined.

We have attempted in this book to illustrate the excessive use of many kinds of drugs as a first line resource for the care of older people in sickness and in health. We have questioned the need for drugs at all, or in such large amounts, for older people with chronic degenerative conditions. Similar points have been made in relation to insomnia, anxiety and other minor emotional disorders. We have highlighted the drugs, confirmed by many others such as Williamson and Chopin (1980), Comfort (1983) and the Royal College of Physicians (1984), which are associated with the highest risk of adverse drug reactions. These include antihypertensive drugs, diuretics, digoxin, sedatives, sleeping pills, anti-parkinsonian agents and minor and major tranquillisers (neuroleptics). We have questioned the price older people pay for drug treatment in terms of the frequency of these adverse reactions.

Not only is there a need for vigilance by health care workers to assess the cost/benefit ratio in individual elderly patients undergoing drug treatment, there should also be continuing attention to safety procedures in terms of drug monitoring, especially for new drugs.

In many instances, drugs now given to older people are not needed because they are ineffectual or because although effective their adverse effects are greater than the beneficial effects, that is they make the patient worse.

Alex Comfort has written that: 'There is no such thing

in old age as a minor tranquilliser; there is no such thing as an acceptable long term hypnotic - the most widely advertised "geriatric" preparation has marked cumulative effects on memory' (Comfort, 1983, p.117). Likewise, he emphasised the dangers of the over-zealous treatment of hypertension in old age with the risk of disabling the patient with confusion, dizziness, nausea, impotency and vulnerability to falls.

Should drugs be prescribed when an individual is symptom-free, e.g. for raised blood pressure, she/he may in fact feel worse when given drugs. This must always be explained to the patient. In addition, if patients are dissatisfied with their treatment they should be free to discuss this with their doctor. The doctor in turn should seek to amend the treatment to remove the patient's dissatisfaction. The concept of 'blind compliance' with an apparently useless or unacceptable regime is inappropriate. In fact, non-compliance is more likely, the hoarding of drugs then follows, with the final scenario being the older person taking the drugs at random from their 'geriatric confectionery', thus making adverse reactions almost inevitable.

Sharpe and Kay have written that: 'The successful medical treatment of geriatric patients has proven to be an elusive goal in spite of modern drugs and techniques' (Sharpe and Kay, 1977, p.32). Despite these considered views on the serious limitation of drug therapy in the elderly: 'Everywhere health agencies have been committed to a primary care policy that involves the almost exclusive use of prescription drugs' (Melville and Johnson, 1982, p.101).

The debate needs to be extended on management and treatment procedures which use fewer drugs and which experiment with alternative or complementary medicine. It is necessary to avoid the two extremes, namely drugs being the only treatment practice for the elderly, or the equal mistake of avoiding drug treatment at all costs. Our argument is, first, against excessive prescribing of multiple kinds of drugs of uncertain value; secondly, against drugs where the ratio of value to danger shifts towards the latter. We have to keep reminding ourselves, with regard to drugs, that growing old involves an increase in the diversity of impairments, these changes vary markedly from individual to individual and are often totally unpredictable in general clinical practice.

There is increasing awareness within the medical profession and within other health care professions that the rational use of drugs in the elderly, and especially the very elderly, is difficult. In prescribing, the doctor must evaluate the medical and social significance of each symptom, because many symptoms may best be left without drug treatment. Growing old is not a disease, but growing old increases vulnerabilities to the response to drugs. These must be taken into account, whether they stem from poor diet, physical inactivity, chronic illness, or the reduced efficiency of particular organ systems.

Better Prescribing

It is important to remember that many of the illnesses or symptoms from which older people suffer are doing the patient no immediate harm and do not require treatment. Certainly, there is no need to prescribe a different drug for each disease or symptom. The decision to prescribe should be made in the light of the drug's pharmacokinetics and pharmacodynamics (see Chapter 2), and their potential to produce adverse effects in the elderly.

There is a very restricted need to continue drugs in the elderly indefinitely or to take many at the same time. Many old people admitted to hospital improve greatly when the particular regime of drugs that they have been taking is stopped. The need to discontinue medication in the old, especially when adding new drugs, cannot be over-emphasised. Much suffering of drug adverse reactions or interactions could be prevented, with considerable savings in money, with the regular review of the need for continued medication.

There are a number of reviews of rational therapeutics when prescribing for older people. Amongst these we would cite those compiled by George (1981), the World Health Organisation (WHO) (1981, 1985), Taylor (1983), D'Arcy and McElnay (1983), Parish and Dogett (1983), the Royal College of Physicians (1984) and Weedle and Parish (1984).

In the case of the residential sector, the Pharmaceutical Society of Great Britain have produced an extensive set of guidelines for improving medication procedures (Pharmaceutical Society, 1986).

The WHO (1981) report outlined a number of proposals for rational drug therapy for older people. It is worthwhile reiterating in brief some of the recommended strategies:

1. Drugs should not be used for longer than necessary and repeat prescriptions should be reviewed at periodic intervals.

2. Drug treatment should never be regarded as a substitute for time spent in helpful advice or in endeavouring to plan treatment by simple adjustment of the daily living of the elderly individual.

3. The margin between therapeutic effect and toxicity is so small in many cases that a drug which is indicated for a particular condition in younger patients may be unsuitable in an elderly patient with the same condition.

4. The fewest number of drugs that a patient needs should always be used. Drug regimes should be easy to follow.

5. Touch and colour vision are well preserved in the elderly, making the size, shape and colour of tablets very important components to correct drug compliance. Large tablets should be avoided as the elderly often have difficulty in swallowing. Liquid preparations are usually acceptable to older people.

6. Drugs should be specially packed and clearly labelled in containers that can be readily opened by disabled people.

7. The elderly patient should be taught to understand his or her drugs. Time should be spent on educating the patient on their use and administration. Clear instructions should also be made in writing. A calendar to record daily drug administration may also be required.

8. It may be necessary to involve a relative, friend or neighbour to supervise potent drugs, especially when the elderly person lives alone and has problems with memory.

9. There must be regular reviews of treatment. Drug regimes should be discontinued when no longer needed.

These are some of the main principles underlying better prescribing habits for older people. The WHO principles of 1980 bear a resemblance to the simple rules of rational prescribing for the elderly made by Hall in 1973.

1. Know the pharmacological action of the drug being used.

2. Use the lowest dose that is effective in the individual patient.

3. Use the fewest drugs the patient needs.

4. Do not use drugs to treat symptoms without first discovering the cause of the symptom.

5. Do not withhold drugs on account of old age.

6. Do not use a drug if the symptoms it causes are worse than those it is supposed to relieve.

7. Do not continue a drug if it is no longer necessary. If a drug is to be given, there must be an indication for it in the form of a properly established diagnosis; the administration of drugs on a purely speculative basis is hazardous in patients of any age and no less so in the

elderly. Inadequate diagnostic effort may well result in a patient being treated for conditions that he does not have with drugs likely to provoke adverse reactions (Hall, 1973, p.582).

Finally, as will be noted below, overcoming the problems affecting drug prescribing requires the collaboration of all the professional disciplines and caring agencies, in addition to central government. Little value can come from finding a single scapegoat like the doctor. Guidelines that lead to improved practice require co-operation and collaboration including that by older people themselves.

Polypharmacy

The indications for long-term polypharmacy in the elderly are few (Jones, 1976). Short-term polypharmacy is sometimes necessary and acceptable provided drug dosage is adjusted for age, the presence of renal and liver disease is considered, and the combination of drugs is looked at for possible interactions. The disadvantages of the increased complexity of drug regimes for the elderly are considerable, and it is undoubtedly preferable to attempt to find the appropriate dose of a single drug rather than to combine the hazards of even two drugs.
    If polypharmacy cannot be avoided particular care should be taken with certain groups of drugs. George (1980) lists digoxin, antihypertensives, hypoglycaemic agents, anticoagulants and anticonvulsants. There are, of course, others; those that depress the central nervous system (the psychotropic drugs) stand out as particularly important (Prescott, 1979). This 'danger list' is similar to the one drawn up by the Royal College of Physicians (1984).

Labels and Drug Containers

In the past, although most prescribed medicines for the elderly have been labelled, most have lacked explicit instructions about indications for taking the tablets, together with dispensing and expiry dates. Many labels have been found to be illegible and many others had the ubiquitous 'as directed' instructions (Law and Chalmers, 1976). With the introduction, in January 1984, of the British Pharmaceutical Society's requirements for large typed or machine printed labels, more older people can now actually read the instructions designed for them. Where drugs are not essential, further details should be on the label, e.g. 'One at night as required for sleep', or 'two tablets four times a day if necessary for pain'.
    A container in which a day's supply can be laid out is useful especially for those taking three or more different

drugs. Various types of dispenser have been designed that allow any helper to lay out the drugs for the patient and readily check that they have been taken. Opaque child-proof containers are a source of much error and consternation as many are 'granny-proof' (Law and Chalmers, 1976). For those who have particular difficulty with manual dexterity, large winged screw lids have proved useful. The shape and colour of tablets are important because older people retain discrimination in colour and shape. Confusion can arise if the doctor prescribes a different brand of the same drug. Treatment is facilitated when the patients bring all their drugs to the consultation and when careful records of repeat prescriptions are made.

Memory Aids

Packaging devices have recently been introduced to act as memory aids, especially for those with complicated drug regimes or in those who have memory difficulties. Calendar packs similar to those used for oral contraceptives, 'Dial Pack', 'Dossett' and 'Medidos' trays, are examples. These devices are only standardising many patients' attempts to devise their own memory aids such as setting out doses for the day or week. The typical tray has 28 blisters in 4 rows of 7 to represent each day of the week. The pills for each day can be put into each blister by the patient, relative or home help and covered with one or four sliding clear plastic covers. Thus they can display up to a week's supply of tablets and capsules in a closed plastic container for four dose times per day.

An improvement in compliance with such devices in patients of all ages was illustrated by Linkewich et al. (1974), who found that the number of patients taking the correct number of tablets was increased from 28 per cent to 88.5 per cent, by changing from plain labelled medicine bottles to a 'Dial Pack' together with an instruction card.

Written Information

Many simple yet innovative devices have been introduced to help old people improve their ability and commitment to pursue a drug treatment regime. Treatment cards for the patient with simple clearly written drug lists, dosage and timing have been designed. A sample of each drug stuck down with sellotape and a brief comment of what it is for in language that can easily be understood have helped many older patients (e.g. 'water tablets', 'pain tablets' and 'breathing tablets'). These personal cards act as a ready check and reinforce verbal instructions that have been given earlier and which can be reinforced in the future. Written instructions increase drug compliance (Wandless and Davie,

1977) over and beyond verbal instructions. In some cases a calendar sheet listing the dose and time of each medicine, with spaces for the patient to check off every dose, has proved useful and acceptable. However, rather than a single method a combined approach using visual and verbal reminders from doctors, pharmacists, community nurses and relatives is preferable.

Finally, information leaflets (Drury, 1984) have been devised for patients on long-term treatment for conditions such as hypertension (George, 1983) or depression (Myers and Calvert, 1978). Such material has been shown to increase the patient's knowledge of and satisfaction with their medication. Information booklets are now available to the patient on a range of medical topics (Sloan, 1984). Not to be outdone by their medical colleagues, pharmacists have also made recommendations on information leaflets for patients (Laekeman, 1984). In addition, as Taylor (1983) points out, the spread of information about drugs to the able and fit elderly majority may be facilitated by the general education of the younger population who may pass on their learning to older relatives in the course of their day-to-day contact.

The issuing of repeat prescriptions is a continuing problem for older people. In response to this, many surgeries are now devising improved safety measures on prescribing. With the appropriate filing card system or microcomputer, the primary care team and the patient could, for example, have instructions that their prescriptions could only be repeated on two occasions. In other words, after this point the prescription could not be re-issued until they saw their GP. Different medical practices have established their own monitoring procedures for repeat prescriptions.

Roland and his colleagues (1985) introduced a computer-assisted repeat-prescribing programme into their general practice. They found that improvements were made in several aspects of practice organisation. Apart from auditing their own prescribing, time was saved by doctors and receptionists, data were processed more quickly and accurately and information in the records about drugs that were available for repeat prescriptions was improved. This procedure can be augmented by those patients on regular medicines (a predominance of whom are older people) having their own treatment cards.

The Hospital and the Community

Many prescribing problems arise from the unnecessarily large gap between the GP and the hospital doctor in the ongoing care of older people. The links between primary care and secondary hospital care doctors should be shortened and made more secure. Part of the fault here is the separate administrative structure within the NHS of the two groups of doctors. Probably the principle that the GP is the arbiter and prescriber of drugs for older people in the community is as valid now as it ever was.

It is well recognised that after discharge from hospital some patients spontaneously resume the medication prescribed for them before their admission, often because the patient feels unclear as to what he should be taking after discharge. Parkin et al. (1976) reported on a follow-up of patients discharged from hospital and their actual drug-taking practices. They found that 66 of the 130 patients that they followed through deviated from their drug regime prescribed on discharge from hospital acute medical wards. Of the 66, 46 did not have a clear understanding of the regimes and the remaining 20 understood the regimes but did not follow instructions. They found that the failure to understand and the non-compliance related to the complexity of the drug regimes and the availability of medicines prescribed before admission to hospital.

In a further attempt to grasp what exactly happened to the drug-taking routines of patients discharged from hospital geriatric units, Abrahams and Andrews (1984) have reported some interesting findings. They first found that on admission many drugs were discontinued, confirming the claim of many geriatricians that they cure as many patients by stopping drugs as by starting medication. The four commonest drugs stopped on admission to hospital were sedatives, diuretics, analgesics and antibiotics. However, they also found that many drugs were later started in hospital, including those in the groups that were most likely to be stopped. On leaving hospital the patients were followed up and their drug-taking regimes recorded on a number of occasions. Nearly half the patients had started new drugs within 2-3 weeks of discharge, with both the GP as well as the patients initiating these changes. This proportion increased at later follow-ups.

When closely questioned, only half understood about the dosage and timing of all their drugs, a quarter understood some of their drugs and 14 per cent did not understand any.

Macdonald et al. have reported on their experiments to improve drug compliance after hospital discharge. The main thrust of their work was to assess the effect of a designated member of staff spending about 15 minutes with each elderly patient before discharge. The purpose of this was to ensure: first, that their drug regime was fully understood and remembered; secondly, that old tablets were destroyed; and thirdly, that other people's tablets were not taken. Counselling was found to be effective in 165 patients who made less than one-third of the errors made by uncounselled patients. In terms of additional technical aids they found that tear-off daily calendar slips led to modest improvements in compliance.

Treatment may be interrupted by episodes of what is

intended to be short-term therapy initiated perhaps at several different out-patient clinics. In such a situation, it is vital that good communication is maintained between the GP and specialist clinics. A clear record of the treatment policy in the hospital notes would help. Further, this should be communicated to the GP, who is often embarrassed that he does not know what is happening when the patient visits him next.

Conditions that need long-term carefully monitored drug treatment, such as hypertension or refractory depression, present particular difficulty. Should these patients be programmed to have continuous monitoring at the hospital, this must be clearly stated to the GP, who has to maintain the patient's records in the most meaningful and up-to-date manner possible. Generally it is recommended that, except for very specific reasons, the bulk of patients should receive their long-term care from the GP. This means that, when the treatment is recommended to be continued for any length of time by the hospital, or if it is complicated, detailed information on the treatment policy and how it should be monitored (and when it should be stopped) must be conveyed to the GP.

The transition from hospital to community must be seen as part of a continuum of care and not as one agency relinquishing responsibility to another. An assessment of the elderly patient's needs should be identified and effectively organised before discharge. To ensure drug treatment compliance and long-term drug monitoring this will involve collaboration between different professional disciplines both in hospital and in the community. Where necessary the patient's written information should be shared with the relative or key care worker.

These developments to improve continuity of care do not negate the need for the initial hospital discharge note, including the current drug treatment schedule. GPs say they need the note the day after discharge. Notes available at the time of discharge and delivered by hand best approach this goal (Dover and Low-Beer, 1984), and are thus available to the doctor who first sees the patient after discharge.

Drug Treatment Compliance

Lack of compliance with drug treatment is currently a major concern with therapists. The balance sheet on this equation does not just include stubborn, awkward, forgetful old people, but also includes lack of comprehension of the drug regime (which can in fact be very complicated), and a positive decision on the part of the older patient that they are better off without the drug. Should the patient make deliberate alterations of dosage him/herself even after apparently understanding the instructions, there must be room for further on-going discussions on the drug regime. Only by doctor-patient collaboration can one negotiate drug use to obtain the necessary commitment by the patient to comply with an agreed drug schedule. Therapeutic enthusiasm must be carefully measured. Some old people stop their drugs when they have discovered that the drug therapy appears to make no difference to their well-being, or makes them worse. It has been suggested that 'intelligent non-compliance' may be rational behaviour on the part of the patient. Initial concern that their patients fail to take their medicine has later led some doctors to become aware that they may have been wrong on occasions and that their instructions were best ignored.

Some common factors associated with non-compliance include:

1. Characteristics of the container.
2. Labelling.
3. Taste and colour of tablets or capsules.
4. Size and shape.
5. Number of tablets or capsules.
6. Product-related reasons including side effects.
7. Physical and mental disabilities.
8. Lack of understanding.
9. The patient's own beliefs.

Drugs with sedative effects often confuse older people and impair their ability to comply. Large tablets cannot be swallowed and small ones may be difficult physically to handle. Many drugs are needlessly prescribed in divided doses when a single daily dose is possible (e.g. beta-blockers, diuretics and antidepressants as well as minor and major tranquillisers).

After achieving the necessary collaboration between doctor and patient a range of strategies to improve compliance in the elderly have been devised. Complete evaluation of these strategies awaits further ongoing comparative research. They have proved a great advance and it is likely that a repertoire of strategies will always be needed to cope with the particular needs of individual elderly patients.

More evidence is accruing to show that, when elderly patients are given additional instructions with a pharmacist prior to their discharge from hospital, errors in medication can be further reduced (Macdonald et al., 1977; Baxendale et al., 1978). Occupational therapists (amongst other staff) have also been involved in training programmes for the elderly before discharge on how and when to take their medicines. The patient is given a supply of medicines on the ward and becomes responsible, either immediately or in stages, for his or her own medication. Baxendale and his colleagues argue that problems can be detected before discharge and drug times changed or the labelling or packaging adjusted if they are unsuitable.

The Role of Other Health Workers

The progress needed for safer, more effective prescribing amongst the elderly, involves collaboration between doctors and other health workers, as well as relatives and the variety of care workers involved in looking after the frail elderly in the community. Regular home visiting by health visitors, district nurses, occupational therapists and related groups can assist the process of medical control (Baxendale et al., 1978).

The introduction of a community psychiatric nursing service, especially for the elderly mentally ill, is being increasingly appreciated by general practitioners. A number of examples of good practice in this area can be found in the UK. One such is the community nursing services for the elderly mentally ill based at the General Hospital, Hereford. At this hospital, trained psychiatric nurses are available 24 hours a day to provide help and assistance to relatives in coping with elderly mentally ill people. To ensure quick response to calls the nurses are in radio contact with their base. Such schemes, apart from their general value, must increase the potential for safe prescribing in the community.

Nurse practitioners are now established in the USA and in Canada and are just starting in the UK (Hart, 1985). More credence is being given to nurses as therapists. We have already commented on their potential role in the long-term management of hypertension. In the University Hospital of South Manchester, a large DHSS sponsored project led by Dr P. McGuire has involved training nurses to detect anxiety and depression following mastectomy operations. This has proved to be highly beneficial as well as cost-effective. Nursing staff have a particular role and responsibility in the monitoring of drugs taken by older people (Cobb et al., 1984). Their vigilance and early recognition may prove vital. Wade and Finlayson (1983) points out that, if nurses are responsible and accountable for drug compliance and the early detection of adverse drug reactions, it is important that they keep abreast of the current literature. Nurses have a responsibility to teach patients and/or relatives, especially those about to be discharged from hospitals or residential homes, the names, proper dosages and actions of drugs prescribed. As we discussed earlier, supervised self-medication programmes could be introduced before discharge from hospital. Nurses should also clarify loose and potentially dangerous prescribing, such as instructions to 'take as required'. The nurse is not only accountable to his or her superior but should also be accountable to his or her patient. This issue is of particular importance in private nursing homes.

The Receptionist and the Practice Manager

The GP receptionist plays a critical role in the community health delivery service, not least as a liaison worker for the prescription of medicines. In-service training to improve and maintain a high standard of service would seem to have much to commend it. One such in-post training scheme is described by Moules (1984). There is a strong argument to introduce practice managers (as Moules was herself). A manager could, together with the rest of the primary care team, improve record-keeping practices and prescribing practices including standardising safe repeat prescription procedures. Drug prescribing policies could become more atuned to local experience and need. Information, including written information, could be repeatedly reinforced for patients and their families.

The Pharmacist

Pharmacists are currently putting forward their own proposals for greater involvement in the prescribing process, as well as the dispensing and monitoring of drugs. Pharmacists claim that they are well trained and capable of much more than merely dispensing drugs; that they can act as a check on adverse reactions and drug interactions, and that they can limit the extent of polypharmacy (Weedle and Parish, 1984). They also argue that they should be able to give patients some prescriptions.

A past president of the Pharmaceutical Society, David Sharpe, called for mutual access into doctors' and chemists' records. Both professions could benefit by such mutual access, not to all the records but simply the medication section. The Society has proposed the development of compatible systems, but still awaits a response from the Royal College of General Practitioners.

Hostility to these proposals has come from the British Medical Association and rural dispensing GPs who argue that it usurps the doctor's role, that doctors must know everything the patient takes and that confidentiality is broken by pharmacists. Counter claims have included the comments that pharmacists already know what patients are prescribed and have an excellent record on confidentiality. They say they already have to check thousands of GP prescriptions for errors.

Professor Sandy Florence, a member of the CSM, has suggested that patients should register with pharmacists as well as doctors to help reduce the amount of drugs prescribed unnecessarily. He noted that there had been a 30 per cent reduction in drug prescribing in one town in Holland as a result of close collaboration between a pharmacist and ten local doctors.

Analogous arguments have occurred in the hospital setting as pharmacists have become increasingly involved in procedures aimed at safer, more efficacious and economical prescribing. Most hospitals now have ward pharmacists who provide regular advice at ward level to both nurses and doctors and, in some cases, older patients themselves. There have been a few initial interdisciplinary boundary disputes but generally this more intimate role for the pharmacist has been acknowledged as a positive contribution. Hospital and District Drug Formularies, as well as joint codes of practice, or 'Medicine Codes' are being regularly updated, in which the pharmacists play a major role. The potential impact on geriatric wards of a ward pharmacy service for reducing unwanted drug effects, pharmaceutical incompatibilities and rationalising drug treatment schedules seems obvious. Programmes to meet these needs in nursing homes have been successfully introduced in the USA (Lamy, 1980b).

A welcome development in the pharmacist's participation in hospital out-patient clinics for the elderly has been described by Hackett and Moss-Barclay (1984). They provide drug medication profiles and a medication counselling service for patients and their relatives. In so doing they may identify side effects and drug interactions which otherwise might not be noticed. They also advise physicians on rational drug therapy and cost-effective prescribing and identify potential adverse drug reactions, interactions and inappropriate therapy. The detailed records of the patient's drug programmes were included in the notes and welcomed by the doctor for quick and easy reference. They put forward evidence that counselling and the providing of written information significantly increases compliance. In addition they provide a pharmacokinetic service, which, for example, offered drug level monitoring to out-patients for drugs such as digoxin. This in turn allows for a much more sophisticated drug dose adjustment and hence scope for optimum drug treatment.

Community pharmacists in their turn have not been slow in putting up detailed propositions for treatment schedules and cards for each patient in the community. These cards are essential for any elderly person on regular drug treatment, especially where multiple drug schedules are involved. With regular procedures of updating the cards, compliance and safety must improve. Shulman and Shulman (1980) reported on the operation of a two-card medication record system in a general practice pharmacy, which they found of particular value for older patients and those on multiple drug therapy. Patients were advised to carry their card with them at all times. The pharmacy cards had additional data about histories of adverse drug reactions and chronic illness in the patient. Drugs regularly purchased without prescriptions were also noted as well as special cautions such as diabetes or special allergies. Before a new dose or strength was entered on the card the patient was consulted to check that the change was intentional. Shulman and Shulman found that most of those patients over 60 years regularly returned with their cards when they had a new prescription. They reported that the number of potential adverse reactions or interactions detected in a year amounted to about one per 250 items recorded on the cards, most of which could not have been detected without the card system. They also found that the reaction of the doctors to their system was positive and appreciative.

Finally, on a more general point, pharmacies have considerable potential as a source for delivering health care advice and material. In Great Britain, there are 11,500 pharmacies to which six million visits are made daily by the public. One pharmacist has observed that if just 20 leaflets were distributed by every pharmacy on a particular subject, that would mean that 250,000 leaflets would be taken by the public (Pharmaceutical Journal, 8 February 1986, pp. 163-169). Clearly, there is vast potential here to use pharmacies for drug education and health education programmes aimed at older people, and we are likely to see important developments in this area over the next few years.

Drug Education Programmes

Developing innovative drug education programmes is one important task for the future. In Britain, such work is still in its early stages; in America, however, some important projects have been developed by health and social work professionals. The Seniors' Health Program, launched in 1975 by the Chicago-based Augustana Hospital and Health Care Center, is one such example. Under the direction of two half-time geriatric social workers, the programme aims to meet the drug education needs of older people in the Chicago area. This is achieved through group health education, local and out-of-state conferences for health care personnel, health fairs, individual counselling and research. The project works through presentations in sites where older people congregate, through community social agencies, and through drug awareness conferences.

Commenting on the project's work, Janet Plant (1977) writes:

> Educating the elderly consumer/patient is much of what the Seniors' Health Program is about, but that is not the program's only aim. The potential influence of such a program, especially through its professional conferences around the country and its research, is to gradually

bring out far-reaching changes among pharmacists, nurses, physicians, and, perhaps, drug manufacturers. If physicians come to realize that such a diagnosis as "medication noncompliance" exists, that, in fact, every patient may be a potential noncomplier, and that a fair, but as yet undetermined, percentage of noncompliance episodes are unintentional, wouldn't they be inclined to write explicit instructions, rather than "Take as directed," on presciption orders? Wouldn't they explain the instructions verbally in simple terms? Wouldn't pharmacists, drug manufacturers, and physicians strive to prevent drug toxicity episodes by developing a geriatric, or smaller, dose that reflects the reduced renal function, slower metabolism, and other clinical differences in the elderly patient? It is true that health education talks and professional conferences in themselves cannot guarantee that the second and third steps of the learning process – attitude change and correct follow-through to achieve the desired results – ever occur. But by building consumer awareness and raising the conciousness of health care personnel to the medication misuse problem, the Seniors' Health Program focuses much needed attention on the issue and sets the learning process in motion (Plant, 1977, pp. 101-102).

Drug education has also been pursued by the University of Maryland School of Pharmacy. In the Elder-Ed programme, retired pharmacists are paired with pharmacy students to provide drug education to elders at locations such as senior centers. The training for the programme includes subjects specifically relating to drug use by the elderly. Students and the retired pharmacists are also instructed about how to provide relevant educational resources to the elderly audience and to work as a team (Lipton and Lee, forthcoming).

A final example of this type of education work, is the University of Michigan Drug Information Program. Lipton and Lee, in a major survey of drug use amongst the American elderly, summarise this project as follows:

[The programme] is designed to make use of senior citizens as educators. The faculty developed a medication review form that is used by senior citizen educators when they visit elderly patients in their homes. The senior citizen educators identify drugs taken by their elderly clients and record the information. Pharmacy students then evaluate the information on the forms, and these evaluations are returned to the elderly educators. In a program like this, the pharmacy students learn directly about the drug needs of the elderly, while the elderly consumer is helped directly, in the home. In addition, by training the elderly, a preventive care dimension is included. Finally, the senior citizen educators become adept at dealing with the health care system and are able to work for improvement of that system to better meet the needs of the elderly (Lipton and Lee, forthcoming).

Projects such as those described above are urgently needed in this country. They suggest approaches and strategies for dealing with drug mis-use, with positive outcomes for both older people and professionals themselves.

Drug Monitoring

Any policy for controlling drugs must include reforms of drug trials and post-marketing surveillance. The CSM and CRM, together with other national bodies, have a pressing need to devise new methods of surveillance, not least because of the very limited success of the yellow card system. Recent developments to improve monitoring include the request that doctors be particularly alert to adverse reactions when specific drugs are used (the black triangle system). The symbol denotes that a new drug is in use where it is even more important to report anything unexpected both by the doctor and the patient. In addition, a free telephone facility has been made available for doctors to communicate immediately with the CSM concerning possible untoward drug reactions.

The Drugs Surveillance Research Unit at Southampton University provides another avenue for monitoring drugs. The unit invites participation from doctors nationally who have been identified by the Prescribing Pricing Authority as having patients receiving the drug under study. The prescribers are asked to provide retrospective details of all clinical events following administration of the drug in all their recipients. There are no controls in this method, but there is the potential for earlier detection of toxicity.

Computers and view data schemes offer huge potential for improved reporting and spread of information on adverse reactions to drugs. The CSM have initiated a pilot project, using visual display units (VDUs), testing their value in reporting adverse drug reactions. The CSM hopes that by using VDU systems to report adverse reactions, instead of the traditional 'yellow card', the rate of reporting may increase, more complete data will be sent, and the system will cut down errors and delays at the DHSS. Doctors participating in the pilot project (and there are several hundred so far) are able to submit adverse reaction reports, amend them later if necessary, to receive general and personal messages from the CSM and to obtain information on the cumulative adverse reactions data on most drugs on the market.

The possibility also exists to organise a reporting system at the local grass-roots level linked in with the sharp end of prescribing practice. This could be at hospital or district level. The organisation would aim to report on, for example, unexpected effects of new drugs in a specified ledger held within the hospital pharmacy, in which every report would be recorded. Regular compilation of reports would be submitted to hospital and drug user committees. The drug companies would be informed and the whole procedure would be accountable to the CSM. This particular practice could be restricted to drugs in their first one to two years following introduction on to the market. The companies could have a responsibility towards the running costs with a set levy towards the expenses. Thus an even-handed record of the side effects of all new drugs, including competitors, could be made.

Another important development was the statement by the CSM, issued in 1984, that:

> For all drugs indicated for conditions occurring in the elderly the product literature, including the data sheet, should contain specific advice for prescribing in the elderly. In considering applications for drugs indicated for conditions occurring in the elderly, the Committee will take into account the following factors in deciding whether it would wish to see studies specifically in elderly patients:
>
> * the degree to which the drug is likely to be used in the elderly;
> * the therapeutic index [i.e. the ratio of the therapeutic to the toxic dose];
> * the route of elimination with particular reference to renal function;
> * possible drug interactions with other drugs commonly used in the elderly;
> * possible effects upon drug pharmacokinetics and pharmacodynamics produced by changes in the function of organs, the physiology of which alters with age or which may commonly be affected by disease in the elderly;
> * membership of a therapeutic class which has previously produced problems in the elderly (Geriatric Medicine, 1984, p.156).

Clinical studies of elderly patients are now required for product licence applications for new chemical entities or novel formulations which may be used in the elderly, if any of the factors listed by the CSM give cause for concern about the product.

Finally, drug firms were asked in 1986 to set up a

voluntary system of large-scale studies involving a minimum of 10,000 patients to monitor the side effects of new drugs. This request came from a working part set up by the CSM to improve safety measures following the withdrawal of the anti-arthritis drug, benoxaprofen.

These developments, coming as they do some two decades since the formation of the CSM, seem long overdue. It must be considered unfortunate, to say the least, that such policies were lacking at the time (in the 1950s and 1960s) when the older population was undergoing rapid expansion, and when drug consumption was also accelerating.

Drug Advertising

Finally, rational prescribing will also be helped through reforming the advertising and promotion of drugs. Here, we support Shulman's view that new rules are needed for the acceptance of advertisements for drugs in medical journals. These rules should prevent: 'the trivialisation of side effects, the printing of misleading statements or supply of insufficient information'. In addition: 'Important information on dosage, side effects, contra-indications and drug inter-actions [should be] in a print size at least as prominent as the rest of the advertisement' (Shulman, 1983c, p.10). However, we would go further than this in two major respects. First, we would question whether the language and presentation used in drug adverts should be identical to that which is used for advertising all kinds of commodities. It is difficult to envisage how even new rules can be successful if advertising retains its present form, with its focus on dramatic visual imagery in preference to clearly-designed displays of relevant prescribing information.

Secondly, a balance must be struck between advertising drug products and educating health care workers about other approaches to achieving health in old age. At a practical level, we think that medical journals would be much improved if there was an equal number of health education adverts to those provided by the pharmaceutical industry. Moreover, we suggest that the financing of these advertisements should be derived from the industry's own promotional budget. So, for example, for every polished advert extolling the virtue of a new anti-arthritic preparation, the industry should pay for an equally glossy presentation, focusing upon complementary approaches in areas such as diet, exercise, self-help and counselling. This would ensure that drug education and health education at least competed on fairer and more equal terms.

Chapter 9

CONTROLLING DRUGS:
RECOMMENDATIONS ON DRUG PRESCRIBING

Introduction

In this chapter, we extend our discussion by examining good practice in prescribing in a number of key areas: hypertension, tranquillisers and antidepressants, and prescribing for sleep problems. Clearly, there are many other areas affecting the GP and other health workers, however, we hope that the suggestions and recommendations we make will stimulate a reconsideration of prescribing practices in other conditions affecting older people. The arguments should also be related to the views expressed in Chapter 10, regarding the importance of a health education policy within general practice.

Drugs for Hypertension

In Chapter 6 we examined certain drugs used in the treatment of hypertension in older people. We introduced some of the current medical arguments that questioned the use of such drugs, especially the value of treating mild or even moderate hypertension over the age of 70, in the absence of secondary disease such as heart failure. The treatment of hypertension in older people should, it was suggested, begin in middle age. In general, it would seem sensible to maintain therapy successfully established in middle age, but not to initiate treatment over 70. Withdrawal of antihypertensive therapy in those over 70 should be carried out along the lines recommended by Hart (1980) and others:

1. When the reasons for initiating the treatment were inadequate in the first place.

2. When control has been achieved with small doses and additional non-drug methods. Here, when the drugs are stopped the patient usually has a sense of increased well-being and no significant rise in pressure.

3. When unwanted effects outweigh the benefits. In the elderly the conservation of independence, well-being and the capacity to enjoy life take precedence over the prolongation of existence. The risks to commencing inappropriate medication in the elderly in the mistaken belief that any diastolic pressure of over 90 mm Hg constitutes hypertension are considerable.

Amongst older people there is a high prevalence of hypertension and of strokes. It therefore seems natural to link these conditions together and treat the patient's hypertension. However, nearly all the evidence linking hypertension and its treatment to a reduction in end organ disease is when the hypertension (if it exists) is treated in middle age. From the Framingham, Massachusetts data, we know that for hypertension, well-controlled treatment carefully monitored in middle age is found to reduce significantly the incidence of strokes in old age. This control includes non-drug measures as well as drug treatment. Consistent evidence that starting treatment of mild hypertension over the age of 70 will prevent strokes does not yet exist (see Chapter 6); however, there is strong evidence that such treatment is associated with excessive side effects.

When treatment for hypertension in older people is carried out goals and policies for management must incorporate the doctor, the patient and the nurse. Each patient should have a defined target or goal in terms of blood pressure and this goal should be written down and be known by all involved in the treatment. There should also be goals other than the actual blood pressure, e.g. reduction in body weight, dietary changes (including salt content of food), cessation or reduction of smoking and well-judged physical exercise (see Chapter 10).

Although there is some variation of opinion regarding the treatment of those over 65, there is probably general acceptance that in terms of blood pressure in those over 65: 'the objective of treatment should be the maintenance of diastolic pressure around 100 mm Hg and freedom from side effects' (Brocklehurst, 1978, p.139).

In the case of mild hypertension, one option is definitely no drug treatment and certainly none on the basis of a single blood pressure reading. According to Barritt: 'Serial readings that drift at or below 170/105 towards 150/90 over a 3 month period allow one to monitor without treatment for months or years' (Barritt, 1982, p.114). Although this opinion was based on the younger adult the principle holds even more true for the older person.

It is important to remember that symptoms such as headache and dizziness will not be influenced by lowering the blood pressure. Simple reassurance is, in fact, far more effective. Hypertension without significant end organ disease is symptomless. In such circumstances the patient has every chance of being made to feel worse if drug treatment is commenced and the blood pressure is reduced to within the 'normal' adult range.

Dunn, reporting on practical prescribing of cardiac drugs, argues that: 'It is not feasible for the practising physician to have a detailed knowledge of all the drugs available to treat cardiovascular disease. However, he or she should become thoroughly familiar with one or two drugs in each class. For example, a thorough knowledge of one non-selective and one cardio-selective beta-blocking agent would cover most situations in which a beta-blocking drug was indicated.' Dunn suggests that 'This increased use of fewer agents leads the physician to build up his confidence in their use and he will be aware of their likely therapeutic response. It is also much easier to adjust the dosage and to be familiar with relevant information regarding metabolism and route of excretion' (Dunn, 1984, p.413). For example, atenolol is probably preferable in the treatment of hypertension because it is not metabolised in the liver, it is effective and seems to produce fewer side effects in the aged and its effect is more cardio-selective (Hart, 1982).

Concerning diuretics, Dunn also points out that to achieve an initial diuresis may require a higher dose of diuretic than during any maintenance treatment. That is, the dose can usually be reduced after the initial period to produce a satisfactory fall of blood pressure and thus lessen the incidence of adverse effects, such as a fall of serum potassium (hypokalaemia).

The Management of Hypertension

Both Coope (1984) and Hart (1982) raise important questions on the management of hypertension in general practice (where most of it is in fact managed), and on the issue of compliance. They remind us that the Royal College of General Practitioners has decided that the main direction of growth for the primary medical services in the foreseeable future should be in anticipatory care, and that one of the principal opportunities for this is in the direction and management of hypertension.

What is needed, according to Coope, is a fundamental change in the structure of general practice: 'to move away from the traditional pattern based on episodic consultations for symptomatic complaints which has no tradition of follow-up' (Coope, 1984, p.881). The primitive state of the NHS records system inherited from the days of Lloyd George makes systematic collection of data difficult. Simple registers of hypertensive patients kept on a card index file, or on microcomputers (Petrie et al., 1985) are a vital necessity for every practice if patients' treatment is to be maintained.

Concerning compliance, Hart (1982) emphasises that doctors do not even comply with their own proposed standards of care. Professional compliance with the various criteria selected for antihypertensive treatment varied from a maximum of 58 per cent to a minimum of 4 per cent in a series of studies that he cites. In hospital and in general practice: 'disagreement as to what these criteria should be can only be described as chaotic. The main problem seems to be that doctors are trained to accept the aim of excellence for the selected individual consultation, but not to respect the elementary organising skills necessary to achieve it for consultations collectively' (Hart, 1982, p.85). Hart and Coope emphasise the need for the delegation of tasks to nursing staff with continued systematic teaching and discussion within team.

Coope highlights the importance of the training of nurses in the management of hypertension, quoting the MRC trial (Barnes, 1983). In this trial, nurses were trained to screen and treat patients who had mild to moderate hypertension according to a structured protocol. They achieved a high rate of compliance and satisfactory reductions in blood pressure. The British Hypertension Society is now running courses for the training of nurses and Coope argues that these courses should be supported by the DHSS. Coope also talks of the need for doctors to learn the art of delegation. Despite allowances for two ancillary helpers for each principal in general practice, the mean take-up rate is only 1.0 per doctor.

Hart (1982) comments that an educational process for the patient is needed, with perhaps an initial period of planned dependence followed by planned independence. In an American survey he quoted, 90 per cent of those questioned were unaware that the risks and degree of hypertension were generally unrelated to symptoms. In a British survey, 80 per cent were unaware of any risks from their antihypertensive drugs (Williamson et al., 1975). Failure to correct erroneous beliefs such as these are likely to lead to a drift out of control and the attendant risks of haphazard drug-taking.

Public awareness of the meaning of hypertension, together with the skill of doctors in communicating this meaning, is still deficient. Hart (1982), for example, quotes surveys indicating that 83 per cent of patients believed that hypertension was caused by worrying a lot, 40 per cent that treatment was unnecessary in the absence of symptoms and 66 per cent that treatment is only necessary until the blood pressure is normal. Only 14 per cent knew that treatment must usually be continued indefinitely. Treated hypertensives were no better informed than those with normal pressure. As Hart comments: 'It appears that in practice clinicians do not transmit effectively the knowledge necessary for safe and effective care ... where such education cannot be successful medication in the elderly can rarely be justified' (Hart, 1982, p.86).

Hart's education process was both verbal and written, including the use of pamphlets, as well as instructions that side effects should be actively watched for and that the follow-up intervals should not be longer than 4 months. Then the patients should bring all their tablets with them, not only the antihypertensives. With the use of a Box Card Index active search for defaulters should be made, if necessary by home visits from the nurse or health visitor.

Despite examples of computer-assisted shared care in hypertension (Petrie et al., 1985), responsibility for the problem must fall on the primary care team, with hospital specialists initiating guidance on control programmes.

Hart points out that the reorganisation of the NHS in 1974 did not unify the service to permit rational planning and division of labour between primary, secondary and tertiary sectors, or bring together prevention and care into a single function (see, also, Phillipson and Strang, 1984). An ongoing monitoring and treatment service would, he estimates, involve an extra half day a week per GP. This, combined with support from the full primary care team, would require a substantial new public investment in general practice.

Recommendations on the Use of Psychotropics

Effective guidelines have yet to be produced concerning the use of psychotropic drugs in the older age groups. The value of sedatives/tranquillisers and hypnotics, by far the most frequently used psychotropics in the elderly, must, however, be seriously questioned.

These drugs are used in disproportionate amounts in institutional settings, a feature which raises the charge that the drugs are used more to fulfil the needs of the institution (usually to cover understaffing) than the patient.

In the 1970s, the call for non-barbiturate sedatives and hypnotics was answered with the arrival of a whole range of 'me too' benzodiazepine drugs, the hazards of which were discussed earlier. However, the boom/slump cycle of new drugs is turning full circle with the demand for non-benzodiazepine sedatives and hypnotics (Ashton, 1984). But it is important to remember that all sedatives depress the higher activity of the central nervous system. Because of this they are prone to reduce performance and produce dependency.

Many doctors, sensitive to the older person's situation, are beginning to question whether psychotropic drugs are really needed. If tranquillisers/sedatives or hypnotics are prescribed, then this should be done on a short-term basis for a particular crisis, for example a dozen tablets which must last two weeks. These drugs need only be prescribed from a limited list of drugs, preferably selected by a primary care team and drawn up from their own experience. Over time this allows for improved knowlege and safety in drug use. Links could then be forged with local hospital and pharmacy practices together with the development of joint dispensing formularies.

With many of the psychotropic drugs we have an identical situation to that experienced with alcoholism. The Kessel Report (1977) on alcoholism reported that alcohol dependency was primarily caused by heavy regular usage of alcohol over time and not, as is often thought, to a particular type of personality. In line with this, doctors must appreciate their particular role with regard to sedatives, tranquillisers and hypnotics. This is well illustrated by Neumann who wrote: 'An undesirable kind of habituation regarding sleeping pills affects physicians: the widespread and strongly ingrained habit of prescribing the same drug again and again' (Neumann, 1979).

The duration for which psychotropic drugs are prescribed for older people needs serious reconsideration. Medication orders should have automatic discontinuation dates. Renewal allows for a valuable reassessment and averts prolonged, inappropriate and harmful administration of drugs.

In the quest to seek alternatives to psychotropic drugs for the treatment of anxiety symptoms and insomnia, it is important to improve professional standards by setting objectives for such treatment, including a time by which the medication is to be withdrawn. These objectives should be set (where possible) by open dialogue with the patient. If such objectives are not established treatment may be inappropriate or unnecessarily prolonged and the patient subjected to long-term hazards without good reason.

In institutions there is a need to introduce a much more optimistic and flexible philosophy to allow older people to express themselves freely and to maintain maximum independence. This will need additional staff, a change in attitudes with more tolerance of 'unusual' behaviour, and more recognition that meeting residents' emotional needs is as much 'real work' as meeting their physical needs. There should be activities for the residents or patients including physical recreation. It seems to be important to face up to some of life's stresses with the help of others and to avoid resorting to tranquillisers except for occasional unbearable crises.

A number of promising reforms have been introduced into the primary care setting. One GP, for example, carried out his own psychotropic drug prescribing audit. He found, amongst other things, that he had prescribed 25 different psychotropic drugs over a five week period (Varnam, 1981). The GP went on to devise a more rational policy for prescribing these drugs, stating that the self audit had produced a change in his knowledge about the pharmacology of the psychotropics. Milligan (personal communication) reports that his group practice is devising policies which should provide a more unified and controlled approach to the use of drugs. As a consequence, there has been a reduction in the number of drugs in use at any one time. This is of advantage to patients, who benefit from the increased depth of experience that is obtained with the drugs that are used. Milligan also reports a policy which includes no night sedation for the elderly and no repeat prescriptions of psychotropic drugs for the elderly without them being seen by the GP. Such developments among individual GPs and group practices could be strengthened by reforms at regional and national levels. One example that might be cited is the move by Staffordshire GPs to appoint a part-time Research Fellow in Prescribing. The aim of the post is to help doctors choose the best and cheapest medicines for their patients. One of the GPs behind the idea commented:

> At the moment doctors don't necessarily think about their prescribing and are often under pressure from representatives of drug companies. What was needed was a completely independent view about the best buys and the most effective drugs available .... one doctor may know enough about only a limited range of remedies to prescribe confidently and yet a neighbouring GP would be expert in a completely different group of medicines. The new appointment [will] help liaison between the two if needed (<u>Evening Sentinel</u>, 21 August 1985).

Major Tranquillisers and Antidepressants

Improved prescribing of these powerful drugs would reduce widespread suffering amongst older people from their adverse effects, in particular from neurological effects such as parkinsonism and tardive dyskinesia. The use of neuroleptics in neurotic disorders or for 'dizziness' in the elderly should be curtailed (American Psychiatric Association, 1980).

Where neuroleptics are used in organic brain disease and for psychiatric illnesses, the absolute minimum dosage should be used and there should be a rigid re-evaluation of drug schedules, remembering that at least 20 per cent of the elderly run the risk of long-term irreversible tardive dyskinesia. Elderly patients should not be left on these drugs for long periods unless there is a real benefit to be observed. Over time the drug should be reduced or stopped, either because it becomes unnecessary, or because with advancing age the brain becomes increasingly sensitive to the effects of neuroleptic drugs. This is especially so when there is brain damage, or when other drugs, including antiparkinsonian drugs, are added, or when multiple neuroleptics are used (Szabadi, 1984).

For control of very disturbed behaviour in organic confusional states in the elderly other drugs besides neuroleptics are safer. Chlormethiazole (Heminevrin), for example, in low dosage has a short half-life and is relatively well-tolerated. Certainly the spiral of higher and higher doses of major tranquillisers given because of developing tolerance or frustration over results should be avoided.

Among the most significant medical conditions among the elderly leading to long-term institutional care are the dementias. Wide discussion on the very large differences in the use of sedatives and of major tranquillisers in such institutions need to be initiated. In their comparison of the use of medication between New York and London, Mann and his colleagues wrote: 'Drug prescription reflects the characteristics of systems of care rather than characteristics of the residents in care' (Mann et al., 1984, p.892). Styles of managing behavioural problems require regular reappraisal. National guidelines and local policies need to be established to ensure safeguards and to optimise the management of this large and expanding number of elderly people with dementia in institutions. The debate between the 'nursing-medical model' on the one hand and the 'social model' on the other must also continue (Walker, 1983).

The anti-parkinsonian drugs as we have seen (Chapter 5) are very toxic in older people and their widespread use, such as is suggested in surveys (Edwards and Kumar, 1984), should be questioned. If used they should be in the smallest possible dose. When parkinsonism results as an adverse effect of a neuroleptic drug, the dose of the neuroleptic should first be reduced, changed or stopped altogther. We already know that tardive dyskinesia, induced by neuroleptic drugs, is made worse by anti-parkinsonian drugs (Barnes, 1984). Likewise anti-parkinsonian drugs reduce the desired effects of neuroleptics (Johnstone et al., 1983). The best hope for those elderly people with a severe mental illness requiring long-term maintenance treatment with neuroleptics is probably along the lines of a graduated reduction of dosage pioneered in New York by Kane et al. (1983).

With many drugs for older people the onset of the adverse effects (like those mentioned above) may be very delayed and come on insidiously. This emphasises the importance of regular monitoring of patients in this age group. It further highlights the importance of the role of other professionals besides doctors, such as nurses and pharmacists in vigilant aftercare. This should be a joint, continuous undertaking with open communication so that ideal prescribing can be approached as closely as possible. In the ongoing care of older people all the members of the caring team should constantly bear in mind the question: 'Is the disease drug-induced?'

Lamy reports that, in an effort to reduce the hazards of drugs in the elderly in the USA, suggested dosage schedules have been published for psychoactive drugs. He says that: 'Even though they are based only on age and the presence or absence of organic brain syndromes, these guidelines should contribute greatly to safer geriatric medicine' (Lamy, 1980a, p.513). This again argues for a formulary for all drugs specifically for the elderly.

The other major issue with psychotropic drugs is the needless use of several such drugs at the same time, except perhaps in the acute early stages of an illness. Using a single drug would help to reduce adverse reactions. For example, in an older patient with a severe agitated depression the combination of an antidepressant and a major tranquilliser increases the prevalence of the side effects of both drugs (e.g. sudden falls of blood pressure, blurred vision and constipation). Here, a single tricyclic drug with an additional sedative effect given mainly at night (e.g. dothiepin or trimipramine) can itself control severe agitation and insomnia. For older people, the initial dosage should err on the small side and then be increased slowly. A time-limited therapeutic trial with such an antidepressant may for example demonstrate that an apparent case of senile dementia is actually a depression. However, experience has shown that unless a patient with dementia has signs and symptoms of a depressive illness it is rarely beneficial to try antidepressant drugs.

Should side effects become marked in the treatment of a true depressive illness with one of the cheaper traditional antidepressants (as mentioned above), one of the newer drugs such as mianserin or nomifensine may be better tolerated by older people. For the intractable depression (remembering that antidepressant drugs are weak and only lead to a resolution of the condition in two-thirds of cases) or frequently recurring depression, inexpensive lithium salts are proving invaluable. Because lithium, like digoxin, has a very narrow line between its therapeutic dose and its toxic dose, treatment must be preceded by various tests of bodily function (for example of the kidneys) and be regularly monitored by, amongst other tests, repeated assessments of lithium in the blood.

Recommendations on Prescribing for Sleep Problems

Goldson (1981) argues that western society is somewhat preoccupied with the concept of consolidated nocturnal sleep, even though no serious biological consequences result from absent sleep. There is a built-in fear that missing sleep will prevent normal functioning the next day. With ageing the sleep pattern slowly changes (see Chapter 5), and it is in this setting that additional stress in life may prompt the older person or their relative to seek medical help, ostensibly 'because of sleeplessness'. Conflicts over living alone, the experience of reduced living standards, chronic physical illness or loss of security may, in fact, be more relevant. It is in this everyday life situation that dependency on regular hypnotic medication can arise.

Goldson (1981) describes in some detail the process by which the complaint of insomnia in older people should be assessed and managed. It is now well established that tolerance of the effect of hypnotics develops within 3-14 days of continuous use, and that problems exist in relation to withdrawal after continuous use. Patients need to know that stopping a hypnotic, especially after prolonged continuous use, will often lead to broken sleep with vivid dreams ('nightmares') and anxiety.

Overstall (1982), writing on the treatment of sleep disturbances in the elderly, has commented: 'Unless care is taken in selecting patients who are likely to benefit from an hypnotic and in carefully reviewing them at frequent intervals, about one-third will still be taking the hypnotic one year later. Moreover, these patients rate the quality of their sleep as worse than those not on hypnotics which raises doubts as to the benefits of these drugs in the long term' (Overstall, 1982, p.173). Overstall went on to point out that difficulty in withdrawing a hypnotic is the main reason for continued prescription. Dependency has been reported with temazepam (Ratna 1981), the hypnotic now being particularly recommended for the elderly. Virtually all the benzodiazepine drugs raise problems when prescribed for older people. Overstall (1982) concludes that benzodiazepines should be avoided altogether in the very old and the frail (see also Comfort, 1983). The most effective cure for insomnia, although sometimes difficult to achieve, is for the person to increase his or her level of daytime activity.

After excluding a range of varied medical conditions which give rise to the complaint of sleeplessness, there are different types of advice that should be made available to older people and all those concerned with their care. Insufficient food, indigestion, constipation, lack of warmth, sheer loneliness and protracted 'catnaps' in the day can all lead to the development of abnormal sleeping patterns, as can the taking of repeated cups of coffee or tea before going to bed, or even cold and cough remedies that contain stimulants. In addition, some patients have unrealistic sleep expectations which may be pandered to by the routine prescribing of hypnotics.

Basically each person has to find the sleep routine that suits him or her best. If, for example, they cannot get to sleep until one or two in the morning they should try going to bed at that time. In this way, it has been found that people can often have seven to nine hours refreshing sleep.

Biological rhythms are easily disturbed in older people, so that education about sleep habits may be the most helpful therapy.

As a last resort for the elderly patient with true insomnia, which is not just an age problem, it is better to give a short or intermediate acting sedative, to give as small a dose as possible, to avoid increasing the dose, and to give it for short periods of 10-14 days (for a specific problem only). Many studies have confirmed that for the older age group the optimum dosage of a night sedative is half or less than half the optimum dose for those adults less than 55 years (Jovanovic et al., 1980; Greenblatt et al., 1977).

It is particularly important to avoid drug accumulation. In this context, the following advice has been given: 'An essential criterion for such an hypnotic is that it should be effectively cleared from the body before the next dose is given - that is, its half life should be less than 8-10 hours' (British Medical Journal leader, 1980). Kellet (1984) advocates the use of non-benzodiazepine drugs where necessary, i.e. the older cheaper drugs such as chloral derivatives and chlormethiazole, which have an arousing effect on withdrawal, and which are especially effective in the elderly where a tendency to prolong bedrest can lead to progressive weakness and immobility. Repeated revision of prescription is required, unwanted effects sought and the drug stopped as soon as possible. The elderly in particular need to be seen with each prescription (or after a fixed number of repeat prescriptions), as programmed in examples of good practice in primary care (Milligan, personal communication). In such practices, Milligan points out the paramount educative role of the doctor. Many elderly people, including those over 80, are still driving. It is, therefore, the doctor's responsibility to warn the patient that sedatives will interfere with this activity. This advice should be reinforced by a clearly printed label to the same effect on the drug container.

With regard to the excessive use of hypnotics in institutions, we have to ask the question as to whose needs are being met. Few institutions tolerate an old person wandering about for a while at night, whether they take themselves back to bed or need to be shepherded back. Often the pressure comes from understaffing. For example, a nurse on night duty in hospital, in particular if inexperienced and alone, will ensure more than adequate sedation. For her, some patients, especially those she sees as potentially aggressive or interfering, must not, on any account, wake in the night. Again, in a hospital setting a duty doctor called in the night to a patient he does not know, seems very happy to write out heavy medication, to be taken as and when required, which has a particular tendency of continuing in perpetuity.

Serious attempts to reduce or stop night sedation with hypnotics in the institutional situation have been made, some with considerable success. This does require a change of attitude amongst the staff, an agreed common policy and continuity of staff. By the time, for example, an elderly patient with senile dementia has reached institutional care the family may have reached set ideas about night sedation, which may have been given as a routine primarily for the benefit of the carers to give them a restful night. If one drug has not worked the family has asked for another which might even be given with the initial drug as well. Such a patient on going into an institution should be allowed greater physical freedom to walk about. Some of the more restless behaviour should be tolerated; in fact evening dancing can be encouraged with, for example, regular music sessions from say 7 pm to 9 pm each night. A hard and fast bedtime need not be set; the patient will go to bed when tired.

The practice of giving no drugs at night has been pioneered in a number of residential settings. In Woodside Local Authority Home for the Elderly Mentally Infirm in Birmingham, the 30 residents all have advanced organic brain disease (predominantly senile dementia), and have satisfied criteria to reach the top of a waiting list for local authority residential care (or assessment for residential care). All the staff, including the GP, are brought into the spirit of the aims of the home. Although there is a more easy, perhaps noisy, atmosphere, all the residents are carefully monitored (including their sleep and micturition habits). In this milieu, the staff report a distinct decline in aggressive behaviour by the residents. The front door is generally kept locked, but there is freedom of movement throughout almost all of the large home. There is in particular a large total area for activities as well as two moderately large closed gardens at the rear with ready access. Regular socials are held (sometimes involving the immediate local community), and a cheerful, informal atmosphere is generally created. Major tranquillisers are used only if the resident appears tormented and then only temporarily. The staff routine is geared to the lifestyle of the residents rather than vice versa. The patient is allowed to develop her/his own daily rhythm. The patients on average sleep for 6-7 hours per 24. They go to sleep at different times, the majority before midnight, some much later. The staff argue that the residents appear to enjoy their freedom of movement even if this does occasionally give them surprises and some havoc. In reverse a restriction of such freedom leads to more aggression and more havoc.

Formerly this kind of management philosophy was resisted by senior professional and management staff. Sedative medication is now eschewed. Over-sedation is avoided, patients do not become 'vegetables', prematurely inert, doubly incontinent, confused and in need of heavy nursing care as well as having to be fed. Untoward behaviour leading to a vicious circle of increasing sedation is avoided. Over-sedated residents may need two people to stand them up and dress them, when understaffing ironically may have been used as an excuse to use sedation in the first place. At Woodside, staff would rather have a resident to chase after than require as many as three staff to lift them up. True, some patients become more active without tranquillisers, but they also become brighter and more able to contribute to the running of their home with such tasks as washing up.

Should they get up during the night the staff make one attempt to get them back to bed. Should this fail they feel that the resident must be allowed 'to do their own thing'. The medical staff do not act in the routine way by responding unquestioningly to a request for sedation by the staff.

The Woodside Home practice of avoiding night sedation invites serious examination, as do other management initiatives in the care of the elderly with dementia. Such an initiative is evening care from, say, 4.30 to 10.30 pm, again allowing the cessation of night sedation. Thus the elderly disturbed, demented patient in the community, instead of having day care, has evening care involving social and physical activity. This and such-like facilities could correspond more closely to what their families need. The advantages and disadvantages of sedation must also be carefully explained to the family members. A night sitting service once or twice a week and relative self-help groups are other potential initiatives.

Another example questioning the need for sedation can be found in the psychiatric service in Galway, Eire. They have created a sleeping, pill, free community in their day hospital, and in a 40-bed psychiatric unit of a general hospital. Professor Fahy writes: 'Newly admitted patients requesting hypnotics are informed of the firm policy against night sedation and are given no reason to expect that exceptions are made. There is very good staffing at night - four nurses for 40 beds, with special nurses available - and that is very important. Very few patients in fact fail to sleep, even on the first night of admission' (Fahy, 1980, p.233).

He goes on:

> Despite occasional threats, no patients have found it necessary to discharge themselves against medical advice because of failure to obtain sleeping pills. Some patients, of course, may secretly sub-medicate on the ward despite nursing staff vigilance, and we cannot monitor the incidence of relapse after discharge. We believe that the difficulties of breaking sleeping pill habits have been exaggerated and we suggest that our colleagues outside psychiatry should perhaps look again

at their prescribing habits. We believe that it is now necessary to define the indications, if there are any, for the use of hypnotics in the management of major psychiatric illness.

He concludes:

... it is drug-induced sleep that is the issue with us. We believe that this is a very important social and commercial issue that has developed this century, but in terms of scientific medicine, regardless of how you define the disease, artificially induced sleep has not been shown to be important (Fahy, 1980, p.234).

In response to such contributions, at a meeting of the British Association of Psychopharmacology, Drucker-Colin from Mexico argued:

Perhaps it is not a matter of wanting new hypnotics - it may simply be a matter of educating the physician about their use. I do not know how it is in England, but in the United States physicians are very ignorant about how to use them. There is often no differential diagnosis - the physician treats all of the sleep-disturbed patients the same, without considering the cause of the disturbance. I believe the education of the physician is very important in terms of treatment (Drucker-Colin 1980, p.236).

Chapter 10

CONTROLLING DRUGS:
HEALTH EDUCATION PERSPECTIVES

Introduction

In the previous two chapters we examined various aspects of
professional practice, and made recommendations concerning
the use of drugs in specific areas. In this chapter we shall
review a range of preventive policies, and the role they might
play in reducing the need for drug treatment. Attention will
be given to the role of diet, exercise, self-care and
self-help. There is now a substantial literature on these
themes, and in the space available we can only summarise
some of the key arguments. At the end of the book,
however, the interested reader will find a bibliography on
health education and its potential role in the lives of older
people. Before reviewing some of this literature, some
critical perspectives will be examined concerning the
communication and dissemination of knowledge about
preventive health.

Health Education:The Politics of Preventive Medicine

Learning about prevention in old age is not easy. In
comparison to the colourful images and 'hard sell' of the drug
companies, the advice from health educators can appear
uninspiring. Part of the problem is the difference in
financial budgets. The Health Education Council's (HEC)
budget for 1983-84 was £9.5 million, a figure which compares
unfavourably with the £180 million spent on promoting drugs
in the same period. The HEC figure is also dwarfed by the
annual sum (around £400m in 1983) spent by the food
industry in advertising its products.
    Even more serious than the under-spending on health
education is the political intrigue in this area, the effect of
which has left the public confused and often ambivalent about
health issues. Reports from various health-related
government-sponsored inquiries have either been held back,
censored, or distributed in a different form. The Report of

the Working Group on Inequalities in Health (known as the Black Report after its Chairman, Sir Douglas Black) is one of the best-known examples. In this instance, the Secretary of State for Social Services, unhappy with the recommendations, allowed only 260 duplicated copies of the typescript to be made available - in the week of an August bank holiday. Amongst its recommendations on prevention, the report urged for: national health goals to be established and stated by government after wide consultation and debate; an enlarged programme of health education; stronger measures to combat cigarette smoking; and experimental projects aimed at removing disadvantage in areas with high rates of ill-health and mortality (Townsend and Davidson, 1982).

Campaigns against cigarette smoking have invariably been weakened by the powerful lobby representing the interests of the tobacco manufacturers (Taylor, 1984). In this area, uncomfortable statistics have often been hidden from the public. In the early 1970s, a government working party was formed to assess the economic implications of a reduction in smoking. Amongst its findings were that with a 40 per cent drop in smoking over three decades, no less than half a million lives would be saved. Unfortunately, the 'costs' of this were viewed as substantial: more retired people and more social security payments, combined with high unemployment in areas where tobacco factories had to close. The full report was never published, and only emerged when a copy came into the hands of the Guardian newspaper nearly 10 years later (Taylor, 1984, p.71).

Smoking remains a key health education issue amongst the older age groups. Around one-third of men and one-quarter of women aged 60 and over, are regular smokers; men consuming, on average, 103 cigarettes per week, with 80 cigarettes in the case of women (OPCS, 1985). Longitudinal data, however, suggest that smoking retains its adverse effects on survival in an elderly population, and that there are clear benefits for people older than 65, who have been smoking for several decades, being encouraged to discontinue the habit (Jaich et al., 1984). The implications of such research suggest that, without stronger governmental action against smoking, many of the chronic illnesses experienced in old age will continue.

Censorship has also been at work in the area of food policy. Throughout the 1970s and early 1980s, various committees debated aspects of diet and nutrition. Unfortunately, vested interests in government and within the food industry obstructed the dissemination of information and reports. This was highlighted in the problems encountered by the National Advisory Committee on Nutrition Education (NACNE). NACNE was formed in 1979, and a report was eventually published in 1983. However, this only emerged after considerable political pressure. The Lancet commented that the food industry 'apparently disliked much of what it read and seems to have got the Department of Health to suppress or at any rate delay the report ... ' (cited in Walker and Cannon, 1985, xxxiii). And according to Alastair Mackie (a former Director-General of the Health Education Council):

> The suppressions and evasions of complaisant ministers, a supine Department of Health and powerful lobbyists are winning the day; and the food industry seems set to continue what a Reith lecturer called its enormous success in ruining our diet and consequently our health (cited in Walker and Cannon, 1985, xxxiv).

The NACNE report did eventually appear but only after substantial portions of the draft report had been published in the Lancet, and after pressure had been exerted through the mass media.

Food policy remains a controversial subject. In August 1985, the head of the team writing the first government-sponsored guide to healthy eating threatened to resign over the issue of censorship. The Department of Health demanded changes in the wording of the document, after pressure from representatives of the dairy and meat industries. The Department did eventually agree to publication and withdrew its demands after the chairman of the College of Health (Lord Young of Dartington) let it be known that he proposed circulating copies to college members and the press with the express intention of embarrassing ministers (Guardian, 5 August 1985 and 9 August 1985).

The Nation's Health

The point of the examples given above, is to show that for the individual doctor and his or her patient, messages about prevention - whether smoking, healthy eating or healthy living - may be difficult to interpret and are open to political manipulation.

Compared to such uncertainties the messages of the drug companies are less ambiguous, as well as offering more immediate relief and gratification. In addition, the doctor can point to only a limited number of trials which have tested non-pharmacological approaches. It is relatively easy to secure funding to test the products of the drug companies - not least from the companies themselves. By comparison, organisations such as the Health Education Council have a much smaller budget available for research.

At the same time, it is increasingly clear that the nation's health cannot be left to the pharmaceutical industry. The United Kingdom has the highest rate of deaths from heart disease in the world, and these rates are not dropping to any significant extent (Catford and Ford, 1984). No reduction of average fat consumption has taken place in this country; between 1974 to 1984 it rose, in fact, from 40 per cent to 41 per cent of food energy (food guidelines suggest that average fat consumption should not be more than 30 per cent). One report suggests that concentrations of plasma cholesterol may still be rising (Hawthorne, 1984).

Class differences in health have also been sustained in the post-war period. Unskilled male workers are two and a half times as likely to die between the ages of 15 and 44 as professionals; someone born to professional parents, if he or she remains in that class, is likely to live over 5 years longer than if he or she had been born into an unskilled manual household (Townsend and Davidson, 1982). Worse still, Catford and Ford suggest that: 'there appears little public concern about premature deaths related to heart disease ... of the population over the age of 55, only 3 per cent are seriously worried about having a heart attack' (Catford and Ford, 1984, p.1668).

Drugs cannot, therefore, compensate for inequalities in healthly and unhealthy lifestyles. Few doctors are likely to believe that they can. At the same time, it is increasingly clear that the power of drug companies and the medical establishment is itself a factor in maintaining the existing pattern of ill-health. Taking the NACNE report as an example, Walker and Cannon argue:

> Drugs and surgery may relieve suffering from Western diseases, but such treatment does not affect the number of people who develop these diseases. And in so far as Western diseases are diet-related, the priority should be prevention, rather than treatment; in which case responsibility passes from doctors to government, industry and health educators, and of course also to the individual. But in hospitals the big money and glory is in high technology; in so far as medicine is a business, prevention is bad for business. There is no vested interest in good health. (Walker and Cannon, 1985, xxxii).

For the remainder of this chapter we shall discuss some strategies for developing non-pharmacological approaches to disease and ill-health in middle and later life. The areas discussed are: dietary factors, physical activity, and the role of self-health care.

Dietary Factors

In many ways, it is, as a leader in the Lancet (1984) points out, the very success of pharmacological treatment which has elevated the importance of finding alternative methods to drugs. The subject of the leader was the relationship between diet and hypertension, and the paradox it raised concerning the lowering of the threshold for treating raised blood pressure. The case for treating moderate to severe blood pressure was fairly secure, but the advisability of treating mild or borderline hypertension was, it was suggested, still hotly debated. The leader noted:

> As more and more individuals are regarded as needing treatment, so the attractiveness of non-pharmacological therapy rises for three distinct reasons. Firstly, because of the unimodal distribution of blood-pressure the number of subjects with borderline and mild hypertension far exceeds the number of more severely hypertensive subjects: the economic consequences of drug treatment are therefore correspondingly great. Secondly, the side-effects of drug treatment assume greater relative importance since the treatment can easily be more harmful than the disease. It is possible that some non-pharmacological treatments carry less risk although this belief requires just as rigorous scientific testing. Lastly, drug treatment of established hypertension may be too late to reverse the risk from complications such as ischaemic heart disease. Prophylactic dietary change could therefore, in theory, have great advantages (Lancet leader, 1984, p.671).

The economic factor is, of course, of considerable importance. We noted in Chapter 6 the substantial rise, through the 1960s and 1970s, in the bill for antihypertensive drugs, many of which were given to those with mild or borderline hypertension. Yet during this period substantial evidence had emerged which pointed to the significance of dietary and related factors in promoting a rise in blood pressure.

The connection between obesity and hypertension is particularly strong. In a large Swedish study of middle aged men a quarter of the fattest quintile were taking anti-hypertensive drugs compared with only four per cent of the thinnest quintile (cited by Truswell, 1985a). The Framingham data showed a 6 mm rise in systolic blood pressure and a four mm rise in diastolic blood pressure for a 10 per cent gain in body fat (DHSS/MRC, 1976). These data are particularly important in the British context where 6 per cent of men and 8 per cent of women are obese, and where more than one-third of adults of all ages are considered overweight.

The likelihood of weight reduction leading to a fall in blood pressure is now well established. In the Chicago Coronary Prevention Programme, amongst 519 middle-aged male participants, 333 maintained a 5 kg weight reduction for

10 years. Systolic blood pressure fell by 7-16 mm, depending on the degree of weight loss, and diastolic pressures by 4-10 mm. The Royal College of Physicians, commenting on this result, noted: 'This decrease can be expected to lead to a substantial fall in morbidity and in the need for pharmaceutical treatment. The beneficial effect of quite modest reductions in weight make this a particularly useful approach when dealing with hypertensive patients' (Royal College of Physicians of London, 1983, p.16; see also Velasquez and Hoffman, 1985).

The role of individual dietary factors is more controversial. Evidence for the contribution of salt to high blood pressure is the subject of debate amongst British doctors. Boon and Aronson (1985), in a critical review of the evidence, suggest that research has produced conflicting results: some studies have indicated that a moderate restriction in salt is associated with a fall in blood pressure in patients with essential hypertension; other work has queried this result. Even where a fall in blood pressure does occur, they suggest, it may be caused by other constituents in the diet (e.g. dietary measures to reduce salt intake may also reduce fat intake). The authors conclude that at present there is: 'insufficient evidence to advocate the use of pure restriction of dietary salt in either the treatment or prevention of essential hypertension' (Boon and Aronson, 1985, p.950).

In contrast to the above statement, de Wardener (1984) has pointed to the substantial research evidence linking salt intake and hypertension. Amongst the evidence he cited was (1) 'A close correlation between sodium intake and blood pressure revealed by twenty-seven studies in human populations; (2) the fact that a nationally planned reduction in sodium intake in Belgium caused a fall in daily salt consumption from 15g to 9g between 1968 and 1981 which was associated with an important fall in stroke mortality; (3) the evidence that sodium-retaining drugs ... may produce hypertension' (de Wardener, 1984, p.688).

de Wardener also pointed out that several national committees and two World Health Organisation international committees had recommended a reduction in salt intake.

In general, and despite uncertainty about what it is about salt that cause problems, even the critics accept that: 'salt restriction may be a useful adjunct to drug therapy' (Swales, 1985, p.414). And the NACNE report concluded: 'Eating less salt is likely to cause a modest drop in the population's average blood pressure. But even a small fall would bring as much benefit to a whole population as is now achieved by drug therapy' (cited by Walker and Cannon, 1985, p.21). The NACNE report argued that consumption should be cut by one-half, to 5 grams a day from the present level of 8-12 grams a day.

The role of dietary fat in high blood pressure has been the subject of some important research. Puska et al. (1983) allocated 57 couples, residing in a Finnish community, into three groups: group one received a diet low in fat (with a high polyunsaturated/saturated (p/s) ratio); group two had a reduced daily salt intake; and group three continued their normal diet. At the end of the experiment, systolic blood pressure had declined in group one from 138.4 mm to 129.5 mm and diastolic blood pressure from 88.9 to 81.3 mm. The fall was greater among hypertensive subjects than among people with normal blood pressure. In groups two and three the mean blood pressure changed very little during the study. The researchers concluded that:

> Our results support the hypothesis that a low-fat and high [polyunsaturated/saturated ratio] diet reduces blood pressure, possibly through prostaglandin balance, in both normotensive and hypertensive people. Salt-intake reduction was ineffective in this trial. Thus, changing dietary fat seems a promising method for the non-pharmacological treatment and prevention of hypertension (Puska et al., 1983, p.5).

Experimental research has also indicated the impact of a vegetarian diet in lowering blood pressure (Rouse and Beilin 1984; Rouse et al., 1983). Other critical components in influencing blood pressure include potassium, magnesium and calcium; a lowered intake of these can all help to elevate blood pressure (Truswell, 1985b).

Longitudinal studies are also beginning to confirm the importance of dietary fibre. A British study of 337 men found that a high intake of dietary fibre from cereals was associated with a low risk of coronary heart disease (Morris et al., 1977). An inverse relation between dietary-fibre intake and colon cancer has also been suggested (Burkitt, 1978), although the data on this are inconsistent (Kromhout et al., 1982). The Zutphen longitudinal study in the Netherlands has yielded some interesting findings on dietary factors. In 1960, 871 middle-aged men in the town of Zutphen participated in a survey of risk factors (including diet) for coronary heart disease. During 10 years of follow-up, rates of death from cancer and from all causes were about three times higher in men in the lowest quintile of dietary fibre intake than for those in the highest quintile. The authors concluded that their findings: 'imply that a diet rich in dietary fibre may be protective against death from all diseases in Western societies' (Kromhout et al., 1982, p.521).

The same study has also reported an inverse relation between fish consumption and mortality over a 20 year period. Death from coronary heart disease (CHD) was found to be 50 per cent lower amongst those who did eat fish. The relationship between fish consumption and death from CHD seemed to be independent of other risk factors such as age, blood pressure and serum cholesterol levels. The authors suggested that consumption of as little as one or two fishes per week may have a preventive value in relation to CHD (Kromhout et al., 1982).

The Finnish community of North Karelia provides strong evidence for the effectiveness of a community programme aimed at diet, weight control and other preventive factors:

> North Karelia is the most easterly county of Finland. In 1971 it had the highest (age standardised) death rate from coronary disease in the world. The people were worried and asked the government for help. A community programme was set up. Everyone was advised to stop smoking, eat less fat and more vegetables, avoid obesity, and have their blood pressure checked. By 1979 coronary mortality had fallen by 24 per cent in men and 51 per cent in the women, a significantly greater fall than the general decline in coronary deaths in Finland during the same period (Truswell, 1985b, p.37).

Finally, it is worth making the point that modifications to diet can have a fairly rapid therapeutic effect - it is not just a question of long-term change. Diets which reduce the tendency to thrombosis, for example, may reduce 'the risk of a first or recurrent coronary attack after being eaten for only a few days' (Truswell, 1985b, p.36). Diet may also be important in other areas, though the mechanisms are less understood (e.g. multiple sclerosis, rheumatoid arthritis and oesteoarthritis).

Exercise and Older People

The value of exercise throughout the life cycle is now increasingly recognised. Exercises for the elderly have had a very long history. Kamenatz (1977), for example, notes their popularity in the eighteenth and nineteenth centuries, where they were viewed as having the capacity to prolong life. Contemporary health educators view the benefits of exercise in terms of improving sleep, preventing obesity and increasing self-confidence (Gray, 1982). However, the research evidence to support this is often weaker than in the case of the role of dietary factors. The bulk of data tends to be drawn from non-experimental, retrospective studies. Alternatively, where prospective data have been collected, control groups are often inappropriate, self-selected, or absent altogether (Thornton, 1985). Again, this points to the way in which knowledge about medical intervention in old age has been constructed: we know far more about pharmacological approaches to pain relief (for example, in

oesteoarthritis) than we do about the value of specific forms
of exercise - despite the potential preventive role which the
latter could play.

Some of the areas where exercise is thought to be
beneficial include osteoporosis (Smith, 1985), obesity (Williams
et al., 1982), raised blood pressure (Blair et al., 1984),
depression (Martinsen et al., 1985), arthritis (Lorig and
Fries, 1983) and coronary heart disease (Young, 1984).
Unfortunately, the GP's or community nurse's knowledge about
the value of exercise may be somewhat limited. In relation to
GPs, one survey found that 57 per cent of final year medical
students did not know that physical training reduces the
heart rate response of elderly subjects to sub-mmaximal
exercise (Young, 1984). Gray, on the other hand, in a
manual written for older people, notes that the elderly can
improve their fitness in the same way as younger people, and
he suggests: 'There is increasing evidence that many of the
changes that we had previously assumed to be an inevitable
consequence of ageing are in fact the end result of years
when fitness had been lost' (Gray, 1982, pp.50-51; see also
Shephard, 1983).

The value of exercise for osteoarthritis has been
stressed by a number of writers, and figures prominently in
handbooks on this topic. Lorig and Fries describe a range of
stretching and strengthening exercises designed, they write:
'to prevent the loss of function which may accompany
arthritis' (Lorig and Fries, 1983, p.22). In support of this
approach Dieppe has stressed that:

> Patients should keep fit and active (and not protect
> their joints); they can be told that the joint is trying to
> repair the damage and will thrive on usage. They
> should avoid drugs, doctors and surgeons unless in
> extremis and should know that there is every chance
> that significant symptoms will be self-limiting. (Dieppe,
> 1984, p.23).

There is some research indicating the value of selected
exercises for improving the mobility of joints in older people
(cited in Thornton, 1985, p.8). But we undoubtedly need
longitudinal data in this area, with more knowledge about the
relative value of different types of exercise regimes (e.g.
yoga, aerobics, swimming and gentle jogging).

Some data are available showing the role of exercise in
reducing blood pressure in older age groups. This has been
indicated for a walking-jogging programme (Boyer and Kasch,
1970); for regular vigorous exercise (Lichtenstein, 1985); and
for yoga (Haber (D.), 1983). Thornton suggests that:

> Exercise in the aged appears to lower resting systolic
> blood pressure and to effect progressively smaller

135

increases in heart-rate in response to the demands of exercise, followed by a faster recovery to baseline. Resting levels of cardiac output such as heart-rate, stroke volume and diastolic blood pressure seem not to change (Thornton, 1985, p.9).

Lichtenstein (1985) reviews epidemiological evidence which suggests that lifelong physical activity results in a reduction of cardiovascular disease. However, he suggests that it has not yet been shown that incidence rates are lowered when sedentary middle-aged individuals decide to take up exercise. But he goes on to observe that:

> There is much evidence to suggest that exercise might be beneficial by altering the risk factors for ischaemic [coronary artery] heart disease. The changes brought about by exercise - improvement in physical fitness, reduction in blood pressure and weight and the possibilities of giving up cigarette smoking - make this an attractive procedure for risk factor modification ....
> (Lichtenstein, 1985, p.344).

There are some data available showing the psychological benefits of exercise programmes. A study by Powell found that physical exercise led to improvement in the cognitive and behavioural capacities of patients in a geriatric hospital, a matched control group showing no such improvement (cited in Thornton, 1985). Haber (D.) (1983) detected improved psychological well-being as a result of a ten-week yoga programme, given to low-income elderly people. Perri and Templer (1985) found an aerobic exercise programme improved the self-concept and self-confidence amongst a group of older adults.

From a critical perspective, one must ask how far increased attention and activity per se are the crucial variables, rather than particular types of exercise. In many cases, limitation in research designs makes this a difficult question to answer.

Despite the unsatisfactory nature of much of the evidence, enough research is available to suggest that exercise has potential therapeutic value with older people, and may in some situations either be a useful adjunct or a direct substitute for a drug regime. Further research in this area is, however, urgently required.

Finally, we might observe that the range of exercise and sports activities being sustained by older people in Britain (Bernard, 1985), America (Coppard, 1984) and elsewhere (Hatch and Kickbusch, 1983) underlines, first, the importance of this area and, secondly, the need for professionals to support its expansion.

Self-Health Care and Self-Help

All the areas discussed in this chapter suggest an important role for individual and group activity to maintain and improve health in later life. In fact, the idea of self-health care has emerged as an important theme among many pensioners. Coppard has defined self-health care as 'all the actions and decisions that an individual takes to prevent, diagnose, and treat personal ill health; all individual behaviours calculated to maintain and improve health; and decisions to access and use both informal support systems and formal medical services' (Coppard, 1984, p.3). The skills involved in self-health care include: diagnostic skills (e.g. breast self-examination); skills to manage chronic illnesses (e.g. understanding and monitoring drug regimes); skills for effective health education (e.g. in areas such as exercise, diet and smoking).

The idea of personal responsibility for health is not new (Barker, 1985). It is clearly the case, as Roy Porter notes, that 'a great deal of healing in the past ... has involved professional practitioners only marginally, or not at all, and has been primarily a tale of medical self-help, or community care'. In medicine's history, Porter writes, 'the initiatives have often come from, and power has frequently rested with, the sufferer, or with lay people in general, rather than with the individual physician or the medical profession at large' (Porter, 1985, p.175). Yet this historical truth is open to some variation - depending on the state of professionalisation of health care and the accessibility of medical knowledge. There are some periods when medicine (and its practitioners) play a dominant role in influencing definitions of ill-health; other periods where they are much weaker. The post-war period (from the 1950s to the mid 1970s) was probably a case of the former - even though self-care remained of considerable importance. Currently we are witnessing disenchantment with some aspects of medicine, with concern being expressed at the power of professionals to manipulate and control health resources (Illich, 1977; Kennedy, 1983; McKinlay, 1984). Some of this power resides in the 'gatekeeper' role of doctors to the 'promised land' of drug treatment. By the same token, it is disenchantment with drugs which has contributed to critical perspectives about medicine.

People - both old and young - want more (or less) than a prescription from their GP. But what sort of things do older people want to complement or replace a prescription? What kind of knowledge is involved? What sort of care is emerging?

A central feature of the self-health care movement is the teaching of skills to cope with the acute and chronic illnesses of later life. Instead of these skills being practised and understood by a minority, they are slowly being passed to the patients or clients themselves. The object behind this work is to increase the individual's control over all aspects of the ageing process: from knowledge about the side-effects of particular drugs or awareness about non-pharmacological approaches, to management skills at monitoring an illness which may stay with an individual for the rest of his or her life.

Work in the area of arthritis provides an example of the self-health care approach. Lorig et al. (1984) report on an arthritis self-management course given to older people (20 per cent of whom were over the age of 75) in Northern California. The course examined areas such as: nutrition, doctor/patient communication, use of drugs, a relaxation and joint protection programme, and the design of individual exercises. According to Lorig et al.:

> The course utilized a highly experiential process with emphasis on decision-making. For example, participants were not given specific exercises but instead were taught principles for designing an exercise program. Rather than discuss the evils of arthritis quackery, participants were taught how to evaluate what they read in the popular press and how to make judgements about new treatments. The techniques of group discussion, brainstorming, demonstration, and verbal contracting were used extensively throughout the course. (Lorig et al., 1984, p.456).

Coppard (1984) describes the 'Growing Younger Program' in Boise, Idaho, which has focused upon doctor-patient communication and practising self-diagnosis skills. Over 1,500 neighbourhood groups in Boise have been exposed to the programme over the past 3 years, and it is beginning to reach more frail elderly as well as fitter senior citizens.

The 'Healthy Lifestyles for Seniors' project, another American development, had a number of goals aimed at improving older people's control over their health. Savo (1984), in her monograph on self-care and self-help, summarises these goals as to: (1) increase participants' knowledge of the normal physiological and psychological processes of ageing and the adaptations required by these normal changes; (2) increase participants' positive feelings and attitudes about the ageing process and their ability to make positive lifestyle changes; (3) increase the incidence of participants' accepting responsibility and taking action to improve and maintain their health; and (4) improve measurable indicators of health. Some of the objectives were normalised weight and blood pressure; increased strength, flexibility and feelings of relaxation; and decreased physical pain, stress symptoms and muscle tension.

Evaluation of the programme included pre- and post-intervention data as well as on-going monitoring of the participants' health status. Health measurements taken at the end of the six-month programme, revealed the following:

> The majority of individuals who needed to lose excess weight were able to do so; the average weight loss for these individuals was 12 pounds. A few individuals were able to reduce their blood pressure and/or, under the supervision of the program nurse and their personal physicians, reduce their intake of blood pressure and other medications. A number of dietary variables were improved: a decrease in intake of fat, an increase in the use of whole grains, a decrease in refined sugars and refined foods in general, a decrease in intake of salt and caffeine, a decrease in protein derived from meat, and an increase in use of vegetables and fruits - especially fresh ones - were reported by the majority of program participants (cited in Savo, 1984, p.20).

Work in the area of self-health care is beginning to emerge in Britain (see Glendenning, 1985), particularly under the influence of organisations such as the Health Education Council, Pensioners Link, the Beth Johnson Foundation and Age Concern. However, systematic evaluation of programmes is often lacking. In addition, feedback of results to lay and professional practice is often deficient.

Self-Help and Older People

The idea of self-care is, as we have seen, slowly recovering lost ground amongst the elderly population. The same point can be made of self-help activity, i.e. groups of individuals sharing similar health and social problems. This area has expanded considerably in a variety of countries over the past decade (Hatch and Kichsbuch, 1984). Amongst older people we find: widows' support groups; self-help groups for carers of people with Alzheimer's disease; hypertension clubs; menopause support groups and pensioner health and sports clubs. There is some evidence to suggest that such 'social support' groups can increase the individual's knowledge about his or her disease, enhance self-conception and improve clinical outcomes.[1]

An example of a blood pressure group (in Zagreb) is provided by Lafaille:

> There are two parts to the meeting of the group. In the first part, both blood pressure and weight are recorded. This enables the noting of developments and changes, and individuals can find out which factors are influences on blood pressure. In the second part, the influences on blood pressure are discussed. The

information for such discussion are recorded by the members themselves. So the members talk to each other about their way of life and try to find the connection between factors causing high blood pressure and the blood pressure of each member of the group (Lafaille, 1984, p.173).

Riessman et al. (1984) describe an arthritis clinic in New York which uses self-help techniques. They write:

The Arthritis Clinic at the Downstate Medical Center in Brooklyn, New York, operates a self-help project for its patients. Group members share their experiences and focus on ways to cope with the problems of living and dealing with families, jobs, neighbors, and physical incapacitation. Some of the most important skills discussed are how and when to ask for help (and how to ask people not to help when help is not required); how to question doctors and nurses; and how to perform the exercises patients have developed for themselves. A social network has developed outside the meetings, with members calling each other frequently and planning activities together (Riessman, et al., 1984, p.20).

Riessmann et al. highlight a number of criticisms that have been made of the self-help approach: that it involves blaming the victim; that it diverts attention from basic structural change; and that it fragments problems. However, this article (along with many others, e.g. Macfadyen, 1985) also identifies many positive features of both self-help and self-health care. Such activity can raise consciousness about the inadequacy of existing health resources; increase confidence when dealing with health (and welfare) professionals; assist in combating iatrogenic disease; and widen the scope and effectiveness of health education. In addition, it can help to demystify the nature of the ageing process, revealing it to be a natural and positive feature of the life-cycle. This realisation may also allow individuals to place the role of drugs and other medical interventions into their proper perspective: namely, that they are just one element in a range of strategies for experiencing a healthy old age.

Conclusion

In this chapter we have tried to indicate to the reader a number of non-pharmacological approaches to preventing or managing illnesses which are experienced in later life. Many others could have been mentioned. The range of initiatives currently being taken, in the fields of nutrition, exercise, self-care and self-help, indicate the possibilities for complementing and reducing (in some cases) drug treatment. However, for this possibility to be realised a higher priority must be given to health education and health promotion, particularly amongst people in mid and later life. The disparity in budgets for health promotion as opposed to drug promotion, is considerable. Over the next five years there must be a redressing of the balance, with health and social care professionals, informal carers and older people working together to promote effective health education policies. The Health Education Council's Age Well Campaign will be an important stimulus to this task, but it will need to be strengthened by a major commitment from professionals in the health and social services.[2] In the final chapter we shall relate work in the area of prevention to broader trends currently influencing debates in the area of health and old age.

Footnotes

1. This area is discussed by Stahl and Potts (1985).
2. For a statement of the philosophy behind this programme, see Health Education Council (1985).

Chapter 11

DRUGS AND OLDER PEOPLE: FUTURE PERSPECTIVES

Introduction

This study has tried to develop a critical perspective on the use of drugs in old age. We have presented a dual sociological and pharmacological approach, highlighting deficiencies both in medical practice and in the marketing policies of pharmaceutical companies. If our analysis is accepted, then it is also clear that the problems described will loom even larger in medical debates over the next few years. The reasons for this are not hard to find. First, there is to be a continuing increase in the group who are most vulnerable to the problems we have described: namely, the population of very elderly people (i.e. those aged 75 and over). Secondly, the financial pressures on drug companies will lead to a continuing search both to extend existing markets and to discover new areas of need. This is likely to mean, for older people, a continued emphasis on pharmacological solutions to problems which are social in origin; or, alternatively, the substitution of drugs for an effective policy of health education and prevention (see Chapter 10). Thirdly, the policy of community care and de-institutionalisation will, if carried out (as seems likely) without a major infusion of resources, lead to the pacification of older people in their own homes; this will be achieved through a combination of over-prescribing and under-provision (and under-utilisation) of community nursing and social services staff.

This book has already suggested a number of recommendations for controlling the use of drugs; however, these proposals need to be located within a broader strategy, aimed at older people, together with professional and voluntary workers and informal carers. In developing this strategy, we think that lessons can be drawn from debates within the women's health movement in the 1960s and 1970s. Indeed, as we indicate below, it is likely that the discussions on health issues in old age will follow a very similar path to that taken by women's organisations. For the remainder of this chapter we shall highlight the substance of those debates amongst women, and indicate how they suggest a new framework for identifying priorities and perspectives for old age.

Women and Health Issues

Lesley Doyal (1983) has identified a number of distinct phases in the recent history of the women's health movement. The first phase (during the 1960s and early 1970s) focused upon the problems women faced as consumers of medical care, with particular attention being paid to the question of reproductive technology. There were also in this period, according to Doyal, attempts to redefine existing health perspectives about women. There was a concern:

> to replace the medical view of women as inferior and 'sickly' creatures, with a recognition of their status as normal, healthy human beings. This entailed exposing and struggling against sexist beliefs and practices in medical care. At the same time, there was a growing awareness that certain areas of knowledge that had previously been monopolised by doctors were potentially of immense value to women - knowledge about how our bodies work for example. Systematic efforts were therefore made to demystify medical knowledge and to make it more widely available (Doyal, 1983, p.22).

The second phase of the women's health movement, during the 1970s and early 1980s, saw action to defend the NHS against expenditure cuts and privatisation. There was also, in this period, an attempt to link together the position of women in a capitalist society with their experience of health care and support. This has involved, among other things, an analysis of how medical knowledge and medical practice help to sustain gender divisions within society.

The third phase of the women's health movement has seen the emergence of a radical epidemiology, which has focused on the social production of ill-health amongst women. In practical terms, according to Doyal, this has meant: 'campaigns to improve the living and working conditions of women, and a greater degree of co-operation between sections of the women's health movement and other groups with similar goals' (Doyal, 1983, p.27).

These phases in the women's health movement provide, we would argue, a useful framework for understanding current issues in the area of health and old age. In fact, traces of all three can be found in debates about ageing at the present time. First, there is the struggle to define growing old as a normal part of the life-cycle, with ageing itself being viewed as a positive and healthy experience. Running alongside this perspective is an appreciation that people can exert more control over the quality of their life in old age, through a combination of self-care (individual activities), self-help (group activities), statutory support, and political empowerment (Savo, 1984; Phillipson and Strang, 1984; Bornat et al., 1985; Health Education Council, 1985).

This 'normalisation' of old age is marked, however, by a number of contradictions. For example, the struggle to define growing old as a positive experience has to be set against those economic and political trends which lead to old age being experienced as a form of dependency (Estes, 1979). Alongside a more positive view of ageing, there is a questioning of the excessive use of drugs, particularly as a substitute for structural and political change. With the experience of dependency, on the other hand, the appetite for drugs may be strengthened.

The struggle to 'normalise' ageing is further complicated, at the present time, by the struggle to protect existing statutory health and social services. Evidence from national and regional studies of health services (Iliffe, 1985; British Medical Association, 1986; Greater London Council, 1985; National Union of Public Employees, 1985) and social services (Walker, 1985) indicate, first, the failure to maintain manpower targets for key groups such as health visitors, home helps, physiotherapists and related community personnel; secondly, a shortage of day places and hospital beds, and an expansion in hospital waiting lists, particularly for operations such as hip replacements. Resource shortages in these areas will invariably mean greater difficulties in achieving effective rehabilitation, with an inevitable spiral in the number of patients requiring extensive and permanent medication.

This struggle for resources is likely to involve the politicisation of groups of older people (and those involved in supporting them), who may, hitherto, have accepted the existing distribution and organisation of welfare and health services. In terms of parallels with the women's movement, we might see, for example, campaigns to 'save' services for the elderly which are threatened by cuts (this is, of course, already happening in some areas). We might also envisage the emergence within the caring professions of radical geriatricians, health visitors, social workers, district nurses, etc., developing alternatives to current modes of medical practice within the NHS.

The final parallel with the women's health movement is the development, since the late 1970s, of a radical epidemiology, focusing upon the social creation of sickness and dependency within a capitalist society. In America, the work of Carroll Estes et al. (1984) has highlighted, for example, the linkages between social class and health in old age; and a similar perspective has been illustrated in Britain by documents such as the Black report (Townsend and Davidson, 1982). American data confirm that: 'lower class predicts shorter life expectancy and higher death rates from all diseases' (Estes et al., 1984, p.77); similarly: 'Activity limitation accompanying chronic conditions is greater for those in lower-income and lower-education groups, and for those who are non-white' (Estes et al., 1984, p.81). In Britain, the Black report concluded, in its review of class factors in old age, that:

> The bodies of men seem to exhibit the effects of wear and tear sooner than those of women and those of manual workers sooner than those of non-manual, and the manifestations of degeneration in disease become more frequent. What has to be remembered is that these outcomes are the end product of inequalities in the use made of, and the demands upon, the human body earlier in the lifetime and the kind of environment in which human beings have been placed ... But inequalities in health at the end of the lifetime also emanate from the distribution of rewards associated with the social division of labour. Old age is a time of poverty, albeit poverty expressed in the form of relative deprivation, which among Britain's aged can mean material scarcity in very real terms, as deaths from hypothermia among the old reveal in severe winters ... In old age the relationship between income and the capacity to protect personal health is stronger perhaps than at any other time in the life-cycle, and in general it is likely that individuals who are well endowed through generous or index-linked pension schemes will lead the healthiest, the most comfortable and the longest lives after retirement (Townsend and Davidson, 1982, pp.132-133).

These epidemiological data suggest that social class is also likely to be an important factor in determining patterns of drug use, with low income groups being particularly vulnerable to multiple prescribing.

Towards a Preventive Gerontology

The above arguments have a number of implications for developing a radical health perspective for old age. First, we need campaigns to popularise the idea of a healthy old age, with clearer perspectives for older people on how they can influence - by their own actions - the process of growing old. Secondly, there must be a continuing struggle both to defend and extend the National Health Service. In particular, greater emphasis must be placed on preventive services, aimed at children, adolescents, and people in middle age. Alongside this, there must be improved models of training for paid carers involved with older people. Such models must approach ageing as a social as well as a biological construction; they must identify the patterns of growth in old age, in addition to problems of mental and/or physical decline; and they must instruct students about the impact of ageist beliefs in care settings.

Thirdly, insights from a radical epidemiology can be used to illustrate how the problems affecting older people arise from the cumulative effect of class, gender, and ethnic inequalities through the life-cycle. These inequalities provide the basis for a substantial part of the demand for pharmaceutical products. They also interact with social and class differences in beliefs about longevity itself. These various elements can often lead, particularly for working-class men and women, to feelings of dependency. It is under these conditions that the drug companies find a ready market for their products. The promise of drug therapy is to offer a reprieve from the worst side effects of ageing. When all else has failed or, to be more accurate, before anything else is tried, drugs come to our rescue. One outcome of this is the 'invasion' and 'capture' of many crucial elements of the experience of ageing. By this we mean that people's understanding of how they are growing old is often inseparable from what a number of drugs are doing to their old age. Ageing has been taken over by those who define it as a technical issue, constituting a set of discrete conditions for which there is an appropriate medical response. The idea of controlling and directing our own ageing is largely foreign to our culture, and partly explains our vulnerability to the short-cuts offered by many drugs. They allow us to absent ourselves from influencing the process of ageing, leaving it in the hands of specialists and 'miracle workers' in research laboratories. Unfortunately, disappointment often accompanies faith in the powers of drug therapy, and people are led to unrealistic expectations by the claims and assertions of manufacturers. Faced with this situation, the time has come, we believe, for a massive programme of education about the claims and promises of the drug companies. Older people, as the biggest consumers of drugs, must be a key group in this educative process. If professionals, and other workers and carers, fail to develop campaigns on drug awareness and drug use, then the spiral of suffering from the over-zealous use of drugs will continue.

Alongide this process it will also be important to develop a model of health care which goes beyond the current limitations of geriatric medicine, with its major concern for rehabilitation (Thompson, 1986). Instead, we need to explore the linking of geriatric medicine with gerontology (the study of the ageing process). Hazzard (1983) sees the outcome of such a link in terms of establishing a preventive gerontology, defined as: 'the attenuation of time- and age-related processes to the extent that they fail to become symptomatic until the person approaches the upper limit of the human life span' (Hazzard, 1983, p.279).

The development of a preventive gerontology would have at least three beneficial outcomes: first, in respect of theoretical perspectives on the ageing process; secondly, in terms of the range of therapies applied to older people; thirdly, in terms of the relationship between professional and patient.

In terms of theory, the new discipline should encourage the abandonment of the traditional medical model of the life cycle, viewed in terms of development, maturity and degeneration. As Thompson points out:

> as it cannot be determined when development ends and degeneration begins this suggests that the model is wrong. The old model also explains why, in the general practice setting, there is great interest in human development in patients of pre-school years and why this interest fades away when these patients reach puberty. Furthermore, the unpopularity of geriatric care is understandable, for who wishes to look after patients who are degenerating? (Thompson, 1986, p.30).

Thompson goes on to reject the 'socially unacceptable' term 'ageing', suggesting, instead, that we should think in terms of development proceeding to the end of life, albeit at a slower rate than at other periods of life, such as puberty. This developmental model offers a theoretical base for radical preventive strategies through the life cycle. Secondly, and running alongside this theoretical perspective, a preventive gerontology would support an extension in the range of therapeutic measures to assist older people. This may entail a variety of approaches coming within the framework of complementary medicine, or the employment of a range of health education strategies, or the application of social work techniques (e.g. family therapy, counselling, group work). Finally, a preventive gerontology would, of necessity, be consumer-orientated. Mass prevention strategies, for example, depend upon a knowledgeable and articulate consumer population. Older people would need to become more involved both in their own development through life, and in the services which support them in its later stages. Such a model of provision offers exciting possibilities for a creative dialogue between an individual older person (or a group) and professional, voluntary and informal carers. Within this dialogue, drugs may just be one option in a range of treatment strategies.

Appendix 1

LIMITED LISTS

For a number of years there has been an increasing awareness of the need to control the enormous number of drug preparations on the market. In the United Kingdom there are 17,000 preparations, 4,000 listed in MIMS and the British National Formulary. The increasing number of very similar drugs with almost identical chemical structures, sometimes nick-named 'me too' drugs, is one reason for the huge number of preparations, where each drug company markets its own variation. There are vast numbers of compound preparations, that is preparations with more than one drug, some with trade names that give no hint that they contain potentially dangerous constituents. Identical drugs come out under different brand names, simply because they are made by different manufacturers. Altogether there has beeen an explosion of brand names circulating on the market (Drug and Therapeutics Bulletin, 1985). More drugs are steadily being added to those licensed for over-the-counter sale. The overall situation, therefore, for older people is confusing, alarming and potentially dangerous.

Over the last few years, various official enquiries have made their reports on the matter of drugs and the National Health Service. In 1967 one-third of the most prescribed medicines were officially described as 'undesirable preparations', while effective drugs were estimated as being 50 per cent of the total (Sainsbury Report, 1967). The Greenfield report, published in 1983, recommended limiting the number of drugs on the market, in particular it suggested generic prescribing or generic substitution where appropriate. Such a practice would, it argued, be safer and save money (e.g. Valium under its brand name costs around £24 per 1000 tablets (1985 prices), whereas the identical generic product diazepam costs £1.75 per 1000 (1985 prices)). These recommendations were thought to be financially sound and would also help create some order and increasing safety in the prescribing of drugs. The Department of Health, however, did not take up the advice of the Greenfield

Report, questioning the savings that would accrue by generic substitution. However, the drug industry at that time put the figure at £50,000,000 per year and it was estimated that the system of generic substitution could cut 10 per cent off the total drugs bill. Nothing further was heard until the Government, with untimely haste and the minimum of consultation, introduced its own limited list for 'minor self-limiting illness' in 1984. The alleged intention of the Government was to save the NHS £100,000,000 a year. Following a combined attack by leading medical bodies, most community health councils, the drug industry and the unions, a revised limited list was brought out in April 1985, again primarily with the purpose to cut costs on the NHS drugs bill.

In response to the initial proposal of the Government for its version of a limited list a British Medical Journal leader stated that, 'The proposals contain a muddled mixture of generic prescribing, limited lists and the encouragement of over-the-counter sales' (British Medical Journal leader, 1984, p.1397). To some, the list appeared to be extremely arbitrary, while others felt that it should apply to all drugs rather than a very limited group. Still others thought that it was the forerunner to the further privatisation of health care; namely that a two-tier system would result, with a limited list of drugs for those who could not afford to pay for more expensive 'better' drugs. Of course, most older people would be in the first tier.

The groups of drugs chosen by the Government included those commonly prescribed for only 'minor self-limiting illness'. Unfortunately, for older people such medicines could be crucial to the quality of their lives. For example, there is a need for a wide range of laxatives, especially for those old people who are immobile, seriously ill or dying. The elderly, like many others, would be encouraged to treat their own 'minor self-limiting illnesses'. The parallel process allowed by Government for a wider range and greater number of drugs to be made available for private purchase over-the-counter would inevitably lead to the under-reporting of adverse drug effects. Anxiety about the list for the needs of the elderly has been widespread (Knox, 1985; Oswald, 1984b; Vetter et al., 1985).

Despite this criticism the 'Limited List' has provoked a healthy reconsideration within the medical profession of the doubtful value of some drugs, the value of generic prescribing (or substitution), the need for audit, the need for safer prescribing and the need for local agreements on restricted drug lists. Few would doubt the potential of a limited list for removing ineffectual and unsafe drugs as well as making economies. There is also scope for improving prescribing with the intention by 1987 of informing all GPs of detailed accounts of their prescribing habits from the computers of the Government's Prescribing Pricing Authority (as recommended by the Greenfield Report, 1983). In the hospital situation, selected drug lists have already been devised, incorporating generic substitution when appropriate. This has resulted in the reduction in the number of drugs stocked from, say, one to two thousand to three to four hundred. Substantial savings have been achieved while patients receive the most effective, safe and economic drugs available. Now some group practices in the primary care situation have devised their own limited selected drug lists based on their own needs and experience.

We already have examples from abroad of control over prescribing and the restriction of drugs available for prescribing. In Canadian hospitals, control over prescribing is incorporated into regular accreditation procedures. This accreditation depends on a review of the local prescribing practice and costs. The Norwegians manage on a list of 800 specific chemical entities, nearly 1,100 brand names and 1,900 formulations (as opposed to 25,000 in, for example, Brazil). The Norwegian list represents decisions taken over many years by the Norwegian equivalent of the CSM. The belief is that the drug must be shown to be of acceptable efficacy and safety and that it is 'needed'.

For the NHS limited list to work satisfactorily, there is need for an open debate in the selection of drugs for the list. The committee that decides policy should be made up of experts, independent of the drug industry (which is, unfortunately, not the case at present), including those with real clinical experience in, for example, the care of older people. Patients should also be consulted through their representatives. Selection of drugs should be by cost, safety and efficiency and the procedures for excluding drugs or introducing new drugs must gain the respect of the medical profession and the public at large (i.e. should not be decided in secret).

GLOSSARY OF TERMS

Anxiolytic or sedative drugs also known as minor tranquillisers. These drugs reduce severe anxiety, tension and agitation, without appearing (in very small doses) to reduce the level of consciousness or alertness. They have a high potential for drug dependency.

Alzheimer's dementia is the most common type of irreversible senile dementia. It produces an acquired global impairment of memory and personality but without impairment of consciousness.

Anti-parkinson drugs are drugs used to treat Parkinson's disease or to counteract against drug induced Parkinsonism, a condition very similar to Parkinson's disease.

Benzodiazepine drugs are the most widely prescribed anti-anxiety drugs. They include diazepam (Valium) and temazepam.

Cerebrovascular disease refers to any or all types of disease of the blood vessels of the brain.

Diuretics are drugs used to treat a range of conditions which lead to excessive retention of fluid in the body. They act upon the kidneys to produce an increased output of sodium salt and water in the urine. Diuretics are commonly used for the treatment of high blood pressure.

Drug induced Parkinsonism is a syndrome very similar to Parkinson's disease that can be induced by neuroleptic (major tranquilliser) drugs as an unwanted side effect. It is marked by rigidity or stiffness of the muscles, a loss of associated movements producing various degrees of immobility and mask-like face, together with a spontaneous tremor. There may be other changes such as slurred speech and dribbling from the mouth.

Hyper is a word element meaning increased or excessive.

Hypo is a word element meaning beneath or deficient.

Hypoproteinaemia refers to protein deficiency (especially albumen) in the serum or blood.

Multi-infarct dementia is a relatively common type of irreversible dementia that occurs following multiple small or large infarcts (strokes).

Neuroleptics are a specific group of powerful drugs, sometimes called major tranquillisers, that have an anti-psychotic action.

N.S.A.I.D. stands for non-steroidal anti-inflammatory drug similar to aspirin in efficacy and used in the treatment of various arthritic conditions.

Polpharmacy is the prescription of a number of different types of drugs to be taken simultaneously.

Postural hypotension refers to a sudden fall of blood pressure occurring on adopting the erect position. This fall in blood pressure may lead to dizziness, fainting and collapse.

Psychotropic drugs are mood altering substances which have their primary affect on the central nervous system. They include sedative, hypnotic, stimulant, minor and major tranquillisers and antidepressant drugs.

Tardive dyskinesia is the term given to involuntary movements distorting the face, mouth and tongue. In older people, this condition is frequently induced by neuroleptic drugs.

Vasodilator drugs are designed to cause dilation of the blood vessels.

Appendix 3

SELECT BIBLIOGRAPHY ON HEALTH EDUCATION
AND OLDER PEOPLE

Aagaard, G. (1984) 'Management of Hypertension in the Elderly: The case for "hygiene" measures over drug therapy', Postgraduate Medicine, 76, 61-67

Bernard, M. (1985) Health Education and Activities for Older People: A Review of Current Practice, Working Papers on the Health of Older People, no. 2, Stoke-on-Trent, Health Education Council in association with the Department of Adult and Continuing Education, University of Keele

Bosse, R. and Rose, C. (1984) Smoking and Aging Massachusetts, Lexington Books

Dean, K., Hickey, T. and Holstein, B.E. (1986) Self-Care and Health in Old Age, London, Croom Helm

Estes, C.L. (1979) The Aging Enterprise, San Francisco, Josey-Bass

Estes, C.L., Gerard, L.E., Zones, J.S. and Swan, J.H. (1984) Political Economy, Health and Aging, Boston, Little, Brown

Fallcreek, S. and Mettler, M. (1984) A Healthy Old Age: A Sourcebook for Health Promotion with Older Adults, New York, Haworth Press

Glendenning, F. (1985) New Initiatives in Self-Health Care for Older People, Stoke-on-Trent, A Beth Johnson Foundation Publication in association with Keele University Adult and Continuing Education and the Health Education Council

Goodman, C.E. (1985) 'Nutrition and Exercise Regime that Reverses Bone Loss', Geriatric Medicine, November: 14-19

Gray, J.A.M. (1985) Prevention of Disease in the Elderly, Edinburgh, Churchill Livingstone

Harris, R.H. and Frankel, L.J. (eds) (1977) Guide to Fitness After 50, London, Plenum

Hazzard, W. (1983) 'Preventive Gerontology: Strategies for Healthy Aging', Postgraduate Medicine, 74, 279-287

Health Education Council (1985) Health Education and Promotion Among Older People: Planning Guidelines, London, Health Education Council

Holdsworth, D. and Davies, L. (1982) 'Nutrition Education for the Elderly', Human Nutrition, 35A, (1), 22-27

MacCulley, D.C. (1984) 'Promoting Exercise from General Practice', The Practitioner, 228, 991-993

MacHeath, J. (1984) Activity, Health and Fitness in Old Age, London, Croom Helm

Morisky, D.E., Levine, D.M., Green, L., and Smith, C. (1982) 'Health Education Program Effects on the Management of Hypertension in the Elderly', Archives of Internal Medicine, 142, 1835-1838

Patel, C., Marmot, M.G., Terry, D.J. et al. (1985) 'Trial of Relaxation in Reducing Coronary Risk: Four Year Follow-up', British Medical Journal, 290, 1103-1106

Phillipson, C. and Strang, P. (1984) Health Education and Older People: The Role of Paid Carers, Stoke-on-Trent, Health Education Council in association with the Department of Adult and Continuing Education, University of Keele

Porcino, J. (1983) Growing Older, Getting Better: A Handbook for Women in the Second Half of Life, Massachusetts, Addison-Wesley

Rietz, R. The Menopause: A Positive Approach, London: Unwin Paperbacks

Savo, C. (1984) Self-Care and Self-Help Programmes for Older Adults in the United States, Working Papers on the Health of Older People, no. 1, Stoke-on-Trent, Health Education Council in association with the Department of Adult and Continuing Education, University of Keele

BIBLIOGRAPHY

Abrahams, J. and Andrews, K. (1984) 'The influence of hospital admission on long term medication in elderly patients', Journal of the Royal College of Physicians of London, 18, 225-27

Achenbaum, W.A. (1979) Old Age in the New Land, Baltimore, John Hopkins Press

Adams, G.F. (1965) 'Prospects for patients with strokes with special reference to the hypertensive hemiplegic', British Medical Journal, ii, 253-59

Adams, J. (1984) 'Safety First', New Statesman, 108, 12-13

Adams, K.A. and Smith, D.L. (1978) 'Non-prescription drugs and the elderly patient', Canadian Pharmaceutical Journal, 111, 80-83

Amann, A. ed. (1984) Social Gerontological Research in European Countries - History and Current Trends, West Berlin and Vienna, German Centre of Gerontology, and Ludwig-Boltzmann, Institute of Social Gerontology and Life Span Research

American Psychiatric Association (1980) 'Task force report on late neurological effects of anti-psychiatric drugs', American Journal of Psychiatry, 137, 1163-72

Amery, A., Berthaux, P., Birkenhager, W. et al. (1978) 'Antihypertensive therapy in patients above age 60: third interim report of the European Working Party on High Blood Pressure in the Elderly', Acta Cardiologica, Bruxelles, 33, 113-34

Amery, A., Brixko, P., Clement, D. et al. (1985) 'Mortality and morbidity results from the European Working Party on High Blood Pressure in the Elderly Trial', Lancet, i, 1349-54

Amulree, Lord (1951) Adding Life to Years, London, National Council of Social Services

Anderson, F. and Cowan, N. (1955) 'A Consultative Centre for Old People', Lancet, ii, 239-290

Anderson, F. and Cowan, N.R. (1976) 'Survival of healthy older people', British Journal of Preventive and Social Medicine, 30, 231-32

155

Bibliography

Anderson, R.M. (1980a) 'Prescribing medicine: Who takes what?', Journal of Epidemiology and Community Health, 34, 299-304
Anderson, R.M. (1980b) 'The use of repeatedly prescribed medicines', Journal of the Royal College of General Practitioners, 30, 609-13
Arie, T. (1973) 'Dementia in the elderly: management', British Medical Journal, iv, 602-4
Arie, T. (1981) 'Drugs and confusion in the elderly', Prescribers Journal, 21, 267-72
Armstrong, D. (1981) 'Pathological Life and Death: Medical Spatialisation and Geriatrics', Social Science and Medicine, 15A, 253-257
Asaker, R.L. (1926) Outwitting Old Age, New York, Grant
Ashton, H. (1983) 'Drugs and Driving', Adverse Drug Reaction Bulletin, No 98, 360-63
Ashton, H. (1984) 'Benzodiazepine withdrawal: An unfinished story', British Medical Journal, 288, 1135-40
Avorn, J., Chen, M. and Hartley, R. (1982) 'Scientific versus Commercial Sources of Influence on the Prescribing Behaviour of Physicians', American Journal of Medicine, 73, 4-8
Barker, J. (1985) 'New Initiatives in Self-health Care', in Glendenning, F. (ed.) New Initiatives in Self-Health Care for Older People, Stoke-on-Trent, A Beth Johnson Foundation Publication in association with Keele University Adult Education and the Health Education Council
Barker, L.F. (1936) Live Longer and Be Happy, New York, Appleton-Century
Barnes, G.R. (1983) 'Nurse-run hypertension clinics', Journal of the Royal College of General Practitioners, 33, 820-21
Barnes, R., Veith, R., Okimoto, J. et al. (1982) 'Efficacy of anti-psychotic medication in behaviourally disturbed dementia patients', American Journal of Psychiatry, 139, 1170-74
Barnes, T.R.E. (1984) 'Drug induced movement disorders', The Physician, 1, 731-33
Barnes, T.R.E., Kidger, T. and Gore, S.M. (1983) 'Tardive dyskinesia: a three year follow-up study', Psychological Medicine, 13, 17-81
Barrett, M. and Roberts, H. (1978) 'Doctors and their Patients: The Social Control of Women in General Practice', in Smart, C. and B. (eds) Women, Sexuality and Social Control, London, Routledge and Kegan Paul
Barritt, D.S. (1982) 'What should we do about mild hypertension?', Journal of the Royal College of Physicians of London, 16, 113-116
Bartus, R.T., Dean, R.L., Beer, B. and Lippa, A.S. (1982) 'The cholinergic hypothesis of geriatric memory disfunction', Science, 217, 408-17

156

Baum, C., Kennedy, D., Forbes, M. and Jones, J. (1984), 'Drug use in the United States in 1981', Journal of the American Medical Association, 251, 1293-1297

Baxendale, C., Gourlay, M., Gibson, I.I.J.M. (1978) 'A self medication re-training programme', British Medical Journal, ii, 1278-79

Beeley, L. (1980) 'When do patients on diuretics need potassium replacement?', Adverse Drug Reaction Bulletin, No 84, 304-7

Beevers, D.G., Fairman, M.J., Hamilton, M. and Harper, J.E. (1973) 'Antihypertensive treatment and the course of established cerebrovascular disease', Lancet, i, 1407-9

Bergmann, K. (1982) 'Depression in the elderly', in Isaacs, B. (ed.) Recent advances in Geriatric Medicine, 2, Edinburgh, Churchill Livingstone, pp.159-180

Bernard, M. (1985) Health Education and Activities for Older People: A Review of Current Practice, Stoke-on-Trent, Health Education Council in association with the Department of Adult and Continuing Education, University of Keele

Betts, T.A. and Birtle, J. (1982) 'Effect of two hypnotics on actual driving performance next morning', British Medical Journal, 285, 852

Black, J. et al. (1984) Social Work in Context, London, Tavistock

Blair, S.N., Goodyear, N.N., Gibbons, K.H. and Smith, M. (1984) 'Physical fitness and incidence of hypertension in healthy normotensive men and women', Journal of American Medicine, 252, 487-490

Bliss, M.R. (1981) 'Prescribing for the elderly', British Medical Journal, 283, 203-6

Boon, N.A. and Aronson, J.K. (1985) 'Dietary salt and hypertension: treatment and prevention', British Medical Journal, 290, 949-950

Bornat, J., Phillipson, C. and Ward, S. (1985) A Manifesto for Old Age, London, Pluto Press

Bosanquet, N. (1978) A Future for Old Age London, Temple Smith/New Society

Bottiger, L.E., Furhoff, A.K. and Holmberg, L. (1979) 'Fatal reaction to drugs', Acta Media Scandinavica, 205, 451-56

Bowen, D.M. and Davison, A.N. (1984) 'Dementia in the elderly: biochemical aspects', Journal of the Royal College of Physicians of London, 18, 25-27

Boyer, J.L. and Kasch, F.W. (1970) 'Exercise Therapy in Hypertensive Men', Journal of American Medicine, 249, 3052-3056

Bradshaw, M.J. and Edwards, R.T.M. (1984) 'Do we still fail to recognise postural hypotension?', Paper to the meeting of the British Geriatric Society, Leicester

Braithwaite, J. (1984) Corporate Crime in the Pharmaceutical Industry, London, Routledge and Kegan Paul

Branson, N. and Heinemann, M. (1971) Britain in the Nineteen Thirties, London, Weidenfeld and Nicolson

Breckenridge, A. (1985) 'Treating mild hypertension', British Medical Journal, 291, 89-90

Breen, B. (1982) 'Structural Antecedents of Psychoactive Drug Use Among the Elderly', Ageing and Society, 2, 77-95

British Medical Association (1986) All Our Tomorrows, London, BMA

British Medical Journal leader (1975), 'Tranquillizers Causing Aggression', i, 113-114

British Medical Journal leader (1978a) 'Diuretics in the Elderly', i, 1092-93

British Medical Journal leader (1978b) 'Hypertension - which drug?', ii, 75-76

British Medical Journal leader (1979a) 'Anti-hypertensive treatment in the elderly', ii, 1456-57

British Medical Journal leader (1979b) 'Drugs and male sexual function', ii, 883-84

British Medical Journal leader (1980) 'Hypnotics and hangover', i, 743

British Medical Journal leader (1981) 'Pharmacists as doctors', 285, 264

British Medical Journal leader (1984) 'Doctors drugs and the D.H.S.S.', 289, 1397-8

Brocklehurst, J.C. (ed) (1978) Textbook of Geriatric Medicine and Gerontology, Edinburgh, Churchill Livingstone

Brown, E.A. and MacGregor G.A. (1981) 'Sodium and water retention caused by drugs', Prescribers Journal, 21, 251-57

Burkitt, D.P. (1978) 'Colonic-rectal cancer: fiber and other dietary factors', American Journal of Clinical Nutrition, 31, 58-64

Busson, M. and Dunn, A. (1986) 'Patients' knowledge about prescribed medicines', The Pharmaceutical Journal, 236, 624-626

Byrne, J. and Arie, T. (1985) 'Rational drug treatment of dementia', British Medical Journal, 290, 1845-46

Caird, F.I. (1977a) 'Prescribing for the elderly', British Journal of Hospital Medicine, 17, 610-13

Caird, F.I. (1977b) 'Treatment of hypertension in the elderly', Prescribers Journal, 17, 52-58

Caird, F.I. and Kennedy, R.D. (1977) 'Digitalis and digoxin detoxication in the elderly', Age and Ageing, 6, 21-28

Caprio, F.S. and Grant, O. (1937) Why Grow Old? A guidebook for the man who seeks to remain physically and mentally young, Pennsylvania, Droke

Carboni, D. (1982) Geriatric Medicine in the United States and Great Britain, Connecticut, Greenwood Press

Carey, R.M., Reid, R.A., Ayers, C.R. et al. (1976) 'The Charlottesville blood pressure survey', Journal of the

American Medical Association, 236, 847-51

Carter, A.B. (1970) 'Hypertensive therapy in stroke survivors', Lancet, i, 485-89

Cartwright, A. (1967) Patients and their doctors, London, Routledge and Kegan Paul

Cartwright, A. and Anderson, R. (1981) General practice revisited, London, Tavistock Publications

Castleden, C.M. (1984) 'Therapeutic possibilities in patients with senile dementia', Journal of the Royal College of Physicians of London, 18, 28-31

Castleden, C.M., George, C.F., Marcer, D. and Hallett, C. (1977) 'Increased sensitivity to nitrazepam in old age', British Medical Journal, i, 10-12

Castleden, C.M., Kaye, C.M. and Parsons, R.L. (1975) 'The effect of age on plasma levels of practolol and propranolol', British Journal of Clinical Pharmacology, 2, 303-6

Catford, J. and Ford, S. (1984) 'On the state of the public ill-health: premature mortality in the United Kingdom and Europe', British Medical Journal, 289, 1668-1670

Chapman, S.F. (1976) 'Psychotropic drug use in the elderly. Public ignorance or indifference?' Medical Journal of Australia, ii, 62-64

Charcot, J. (1882) Clinical Lectures on the Diseases of Old Age, London, Sampson Low, Marston, Searle and Rivington

Chisholm, C. (1954) Retire and Enjoy It, London, Phoenix Books

Christopher, L.J., Ballinger, B.R., Shepherd, A. et al. (1978) 'Drug prescribing patterns in the elderly: a cross-section study of in-patients', Age and Ageing, 7, 74-82

Cobb, P., Eastman, M. and Hammond, M. (1984) 'Cutting down on errors - and drugs', Nursing Mirror, 159, vi-viii

Cole, T. (1984) 'The Prophecy of Senescence: G. Stanley Hall and the Reconstruction of Old Age in America', The Gerontologist, 24, 360-366

Coleman, A. (1982) edited by Groombridge, J. Preparation for Retirement in England and Wales: A National Survey, Leicester, National Institute of Adult Education in association with the Pre-Retirement Association

Coleman, V. (1975) The Medicine Men: Drug Makers, Doctors and Patients, London, Temple Smith,

Collier, J. (1985) 'Licensing and Provision of Medicines in the United Kingdom: An Appraisal', The Lancet, ii, 377-381

Collier, J. and New, L. (1984) 'Illegibility of Drug Advertisements' (letter), The Lancet, i, 341-342

Comfort, A. (1982) 'Anxiety in old age', in Wheatley, D. (ed), Psychopharmacology of Old Age, Oxford, Oxford University Press, pp.157-162

Comfort, A. (1983) 'Keynote address', Journal of Chronic Diseases, 36, 117-20

Committee for the Review of Medicines (1980) 'Systematic review of the benzodiazepines', British Medical Journal, 285, 910-12

Committee on Safety of Medicines (1985) 'Update: Drugs and the elderly', British Medical Journal, 290, 1345

Committee on Safety of Medicines (1986) 'Update: Non-steroidal anti-inflammatory drugs and serious gastrointestinal adverse reactions-1', British Medical Journal, 292, 614

Cook, P.J., Huggett, A., Graham-Pole, R. et al. (1983) 'Hypnotic accumulation and hangover in elderly in-patients: a controlled double blind study of temazepam and nitrazepam', British Medical Journal, 286, 100-2

Coope, J. (1984) 'Hypertension in general practice: What is to be done?', British Medical Journal, 288, 880-81

Coppard, L. (1984) 'Self-Health Care and Older People: A Manual for Public Policy and Programme Development', Mimeo, Copenhagen, World Health Organisation

Cornaro, L. (1894) How to Regain Health and Live 100 Years By One Who Did It, London, Marshall Bros

Crammer, J.L., Barraclough, B. and Heine, B. (1982) Use of drugs in psychiatry, Ashford, Headley Brothers

Crooks, J. (1983) 'Rational Therapeutics in the elderly', Journal of Chronic Diseases, 36, 59-65

Crooks, J., O'Malley, K. and Stevenson, I.H. (1976) 'Pharmacokinetics in the Elderly', Clinical Pharmacokinetics, i, 280-296

Dall, J.L.C. (1965) 'Digitalis intoxication in elderly patients', Lancet, i, 194-95

Dall, J.L.C. (1970) 'Maintenance digoxin in elderly patients', British Medical Journal, ii, 705-6

D'Arcy, P.F. and McElnay, J.C. (1983) 'Adverse drug reactions and the elderly patient', Adverse Drug Reactions and Acute Poisoning Review, 2, 67-101

Dane, V. (1930) Grow Old and Stay Young, London, Daniel

Davidson, C., Burkinshaw, L. and Morgan, D.B. (1978) 'Effects of potassium supplements, spironolactone or amelioride on the potassium status of patients with heart failure', Post-Graduate Medical Journal, 54, 405-9

Davidson, W. (1978) 'The hazards of drug treatment in old age' in Brocklehurst, J.C. (ed), Textbook of Geriatric Medicine and Gerontology, Edinburgh, Churchill Livingstone, pp.651-659

DHSS/MRC (1976) Report on Research on Obesity, Compiler W.P.T. James, London, HMSO

Dieppe, P. (1984) 'Is osteoarthritis a self-limiting disorder?', Modern Medicine, October, 17-23

Dovenmuehle, R.H. (1970) 'Aging versus Illness', in Palmore, E. (ed), Normal Aging: Reports from the Duke

Longitudinal Study 1955-1969, Durham, Duke University Press

Dover, S.B. and Low-Beer, T.S. (1984) 'The initial hospital discharge note: send out with the patient or post?', Health Trends, 16, 48

Doyal, L. (1983) 'Women, health and the sexual division of labour: a case study of the women's health movement in Britain', Critical Social Policy, 3, (1), 21-33

Drucker-Colin, R.R. (1980) 'Do we need new hypnotics?', in Wheatley, D. (ed), The Psychopharmacology of Sleep, New York, Raven Press, pp.233-239

Drug and Therapeutics Bulletin (1975) 'Drugs for dementia', 13, 85-7

Drug and Therapeutics Bulletin (1980) 'Helping elderly patients to manage their medicines', 18, 89-91

Drug and Therapeutics Bulletin (1984) 'The drug treatment of Parkinson's Disease', 22, 37-40

Drug and Therapeutics Bulletin (1985) 'Confusing drug names', 23, 77-79

Drury, V.W.M. (1982) 'Repeat prescribing: a review', Journal of the Royal College of General Practitioners, 32, 42-5

Drury, V.W.M. (1984) 'Patient information leaflets', British Medical Journal, 288, 427-28

Dukes, G. (1984) 'Dementia and drugs', THS Health Summary, 1, 6

Dunn, F.G. (1984) 'Cardiac drugs: practical prescribing', Update, 413-21

Dunnell, K. and Cartwright, A. (1972) Medicine Takers, Prescribers and Hoarders, London, Routledge and Kegan Paul

During, D. and Gill, M. (1974) 'Survey of General Practitioners' views on post-graduate education in North-east Scotland', Journal of the Royal College of General Practitioners, 24, 648-654

Eaton, G. and Parish, P. (1976) 'Sources of drug information used by general practitioners', in prescribing in general practice, Journal of the Royal College of General Practitioners, Supplement no 1, 26, 58-63

Edwards, J.G. (1981) 'Adverse Effects of anti-anxiety drugs' Drugs, 22, 405-514

Edwards, S. and Kumar, V. (1984) 'A survey of prescribing of psychotropic drugs in a Birmingham psychiatric hospital', British Journal of Psychiatry, 145, 502-7

Emery, P. and Graham, R. (1982), 'Gastrointestinal blood loss and Piroxicam', Lancet, i, 1302-3

Estes, C.L. (1979) The Aging Enterprise, San Francisco, Josey-Bass

Estes, C.L., Gerard, L.E., Zones, J.S. and Swan, J.H. (1984) Political Economy, Health, and Aging, Boston, Little, Brown and Company

Evans, J.C. and Jarvis, E.H. (1972) 'Nitrazepam and the

Elderly', British Medical Journal, iv, 487

Evans, J.G., Prudham, D. and Wandless, I. (1980) 'Risk factors for strokes in the elderly', in Exton-Smith, A.N. and Barbagollo Sangiorgi, G. (eds), The Ageing Brain: neurological and mental disturbances, London, Plenum Press

Evers, H. (1982) 'Professional Practice and Patient Care: Multi-disciplinary Teamwork in Geriatric Wards', Ageing and Society, 2, 57-77

Every Woman's Doctor Book (1934), London, The Amalgamated Press Ltd

Ewy, G.A., Kapadia, G.G., Lao, L. et al. (1969) 'Digoxin metabolism in the elderly', Circulation, 39, 449-53

Fahy, T.H. (1980) 'Do we need new hypnotics' in Wheatley, D. (ed), Psychopharmacology of sleep, New York, Raven Press, pp.233-239

Fairhurst, E. (1977) 'Teamwork as Panacea: Some underlying assumptions', Unpublished paper read at Annual Conference of the Medical Sociology Group of the British Sociological Association, University of Warwick

Felstein, I. (1969) Later Life: Geriatrics Today and Tomorrow , London, Croom Helm

Fottrell, E., Sheikh, M., Kothari, R. and Sayed, I. (1976) 'Long stay patients with long stay drugs. A case for review; a cause for concern', Lancet, i, 81-82

Gaspar, D. (1980) Hollymoor Hospital dementia service, Lancet i, 1402-5

George, C. (1981) 'The effect of age on drug metabolism', MIMS Magazine, 1st March, 55-9

George, C.F. (1980) 'Can adverse reactions be prevented?', Adverse Drug Reaction Bulletin, 80, 288-290

George, C.F. and Hall, M.R.P. (1981) 'Drugs for dementia', Prescribers Journal, 21, 272-77

George, I.M.S.F. (1983) 'Patient education leaflets for hypertension: a controlled study', Journal of the Royal College of General Practitioners, 33, 508-10

Gilleard, C.J. (1984) Living with Dementia, London, Croom Helm

Gilleard, C.J., Morgan, K. and Wade B.E. (1983) 'Patterns of neuroleptic use among the institutionalised elderly', Acta Psychiatrica Scandinavica, 68, 419-25

Goldney, R.D. (1977) 'Paradoxical reactions to a new minor tranquilliser', Medical Journal of Australia, i, 139-40

Goldson, R.L. (1981) 'Management of sleep disorders in the elderly', Drugs, 21, 390-96

Goodman, L.S. and Gilman, A. (1980) The Pharmacological Basis of Therapeutics, New York, The Macmillan Company

Gray, J.A.M. (1982) Better Health in Retirement, London, Age Concern England

Greater London Council (1985) A Critical Guide to Health

Service Resource Allocation in London, London, GLC

Green, A.R. and Costain, D.W. (1981) Pharmacology and biochemistry of psychiatric disorders, London, John Wiley and Sons

Greenblatt, D.J., Allen, M.D. and Shader, R.I. (1977) 'Toxicity of high dose flurazepam in the elderly', Clinical Pharmacology and Therapeutics, 21, 355-61

Greenblatt, D.J. and Kock-Weset, J. (1973) 'Adverse reactions to spironolactone', Journal of the American Medical Association, 255, 40-43

Greenblatt, D.J. and Shader, R.I. (1974) Benzodiazepines in clinical practice, New York, Raven Press

Greenfield Report (1983) Report to the Secretary of State for Social Services of an Informal Working Group on Effective Prescribing, (Chairman P.R. Greenfield), London, DHSS

Gumpert, M. (1950) You are younger than you think, London, Hammond and Hammond

Haber, C. (1983) Beyond Sixty-five: The Dilemma of Old Age in America's Past, Cambridge, Cambridge University Press

Haber, D. (1983) 'Yoga as a Preventive Health Care Program for White and Black Elders: An Exploratory Study', International Journal of Aging and Human Development, 17, 169-176

Hachinski, V.C., Lassen, N.A. and Marshall, J. (1974) 'Multi-infarct dementia: a cause of mental deterioration in the elderly', Lancet, ii, 207-9

Hackett, K. and Moss-Barclay, C. (1984) 'Pharmacist participation in a geriatric out-patient clinic', British Journal of Pharmaceutical Practice, December, 375-376

Haines, A.P. (1985) 'Catching up the Europeans in preventing heart disease', British Medical Journal, 291, 1667-68

Hale, W.E., Marks, R.G. and Stuart, R.B. (1979), 'Drug Use in a Geriatric Population', Journal of American Geriatric Society, 27, 374-77

Hall, M.R.P. (1973) 'Drug therapy in the elderly', British Medical Journal, iii, 582-84

Hall, R.C.W. and Joffe, J.R. (1972) 'Aberrant response to diazepam: a new syndrome', American Journal of Psychiatry, 129, 738-42

Hamby, R.C., Tovey, J. and Perera, N. (1980) 'Hypokalaemia and diuretics', British Medical Journal, 280, 1187

Hamilton, M., Pickering, G.W., Roberts, J.A.F. and Savey, G.S.C. (1954) 'The aetiology of essential hypertension. The arterial pressure in the general population', Clinical Science, 13, 11-35

Hart, J.T. (1970) 'Semicontinuous screening of a whole community for hypertension', Lancet, ii, 223-26

Hart, J.T. (1979) 'Can we and do we prevent strokes by treating hypertension?', Practitioner, 233, 662-65

Hart, J.T. (1980) Hypertension, Library of General Practice, Edinburgh, Churchill Livingstone

Hart, J.T. (1982) 'Hypertension - does it exist and should it be treated?', in Isaacs, B. (ed), Recent advances in geriatric medicine, 2, Edinburgh, Churchill Livingstone, pp.71-90

Hart, J.T. (1985) 'Practice nurses: an underused resource', British Medical Journal, 290, 1162-63

Hatch, S. and Kickbusch, J. (eds) (1983) Self-Help and Health in Europe, Copenhagen, World Health Organisation

Hawthorne, V. (1984) 'Cholestrol lowering and reducing the risk of coronary heart disease', Lancet, i, 855-6

Hazzard, W. (1983) 'Preventive Gerontology', Post Graduate Medicine, 74, 279-287

Health Education Council (1985) Health Education and Promotion Among Older People: Planning Guidelines, London, HEC

Heath, D.A. and Miller, M.R. (1983) 'Medicine and the Media', British Medical Journal, 287, 904

Helgason, L. (1977) 'Psychiatric services and mental illness in Iceland', Acta Psychiatrica Scandinavia, 268, 1-140

Herbert, S. (1939) Britain's Health, London, Pelican Books

Hicks, R., Funkenstern, H., Dysken, M.W. and Davis, J.M. (1982) 'Geriatric Psychopharmacology', in Birren, J. and Sloane, R.B. (eds) Handbook of Mental Health and Aging, Englewood Cliffs, Prentice-Hall, pp.745-774

Hier, D.B. and Caplan, L.R. (1980) Drugs for senile dementia, Drugs, 20, 74-80

Hindmarsh, I. (1981) in Burrows, G.D. and Werry, J.S. (eds), Advances in human psychopharmacology: a research annual, 2, Greenwich, Jai Press

Hobson, W. (ed) (1956) Introduction to Modern Trends in Geriatrics, London, Butterworth

Hollander, B. (1933) Old Age Deferred, London, Watts and Co.

Honigsbaum, F. (1979) The Division in British Medicine, London, Kogan Page

Hope, J. and Fraser, L. (1985) 'The List Nightmares Come True', GP., December 6: 22

Howell, T. (1950) Old Age, London, H.K. Lewis

Howell, T. (1976) 'Aspects of the History of Geriatric Medicine', Proceedings of the Royal Society of Medicine, 69, 445-449

Hurwitz, N. (1969a) 'Predisposing factors in adverse reactions to drugs', British Medical Journal, i, 536-9

Hurwitz, N. (1969b) 'Admission to hospital due to drugs', British Medical Journal, i, 539-40

Hurwitz, N. and Wade, O.L. (1969) 'Intensive hospital monitoring of adverse reactions to drugs', British Medical Journal, i, 531-6

Iliffe, S. (1983) The NHS, A Picture of Health, London,

Lawrence and Wishart
Iliffe, S. (1985) 'The Politics of Health Care: The NHS under Thatcher', Critical Social Policy, 5, (2) 57-72
Illich, I. (1977) Limits to Medicine, London, Penguin
Imlah, N. (1981) 'Current use of drugs in psychiatric treatment', Pharmaceutical Journal, 227, 351-53
Ingman, S.R., Lawson, I.R., Pierpaoli, P.G. and Blake, P. (1975) 'A survey of the prescribing and administration of drugs in long term care institutions for the elderly', Journal of the American Geriatric Society, 23, 309-16
Isaacs, B. (1981) 'Ageing and the Doctor', in Hobman, D. (ed), The Impact of Ageing: Strategies for Care, London, Croom Helm
Jackson, G., Mahon, W., Pierscianowski, T.A. and Codon, J. (1976) 'Inappropriate antihypertensive therapy in the elderly', Lancet, ii, 1317-18
Jacoby, R.J. (1981) 'Depression in the elderly', British Journal of Hospital Medicine, January, 40-47
Jaich, C., Ostfield, A.M., Freeman, D.H. (1984) 'Smoking and Coronary Heart Disease Mortality in the Elderly', Journal of the American Medical Association, 252, 2831-2834
James, I. (1976) 'Prescribing for the elderly: why it is best to keep it simple', Modern Geriatrics, October, 25-27
James, I. (1978) 'Drugs for anxiety states', Modern Geriatrics, 8, 57-62
Jarvis, E.H. (1981) 'Drugs and the elderly patient', Adverse Drug Reaction Bulletin, No. 86, 312-15
Jeffrey, C. (1939) Fit After Forty, London, Frederick Miller
Johnston, W.J. and McDevitt, D.G. (1979) 'Is maintenance digoxin necessary in patients with sinus rhythm?', Lancet, i, 567-70
Johnstone, E.C., Crow, T.J., Ferrier, I.N. et al. (1983) 'Adverse effects of anti-cholinergic medication on positive schizophrenic symptoms', Psychological Medicine, 13, 512-527
Jones, C.R. (1976) 'Polypharmacy in the Elderly', Geriatric Medicine Update, October, 845-49
Jones, D.A., Sweetnam, P., and Elwood, P.C. (1980) 'Drug prescribing by GPs in Wales and in England', Journal of Epidemiology and Community Health, 34, 119-123
Jones, D.I.R. (1977) 'Self poisoning with drugs: the past twenty years in Sheffield', British Medical Journal, i, 28-29
Jovanovic, U.J., Ott, H., Heidrich, H. et al. (1980) 'Age specific dose of lormetazepam as a night sedative in cases of chronic sleep disturbances', Waking and Sleeping, 4, 223-35
Kales, A., Bixler, E.O., Tan, T.L. et al. (1974) 'Chronic hypnotic drug use: ineffectiveness, drug withdrawal,

insomnia and independence', Journal of the American Medical Association, 227, 513-17

Kales, A., Soldates, C.R., Bixler, E.O. and Kales, J.D. (1983) Early morning insomnia, Science, 220, 95-97

Kamenatz, H.L. (1977) 'History of Exercise for the Elderly' in Harris, R.H. and Frankel, L.J. (eds) Guide to Fitness After 50, London, Plenum, pp.13-33

Kane, J.M., Riffkin, A., Woerner, M. et al. (1983) 'Low dose neuroleptic treatment of outpatient schizophrenics', Archives of General Psychiatry, 40, 893-96

Kane, J.M. and Smith, J. (1982) 'Tardive dyskinesia prevalence and risk factors 1959 to 1979', Archives of General Psychiatry, 39, 473-81

Kannel, W.B., Dawber, T.R., Sorlie, P. and Wolfe, P.A. (1976) 'Components of blood pressure and the risk of atherothrombotic brain infarction': The Framingham study, Stroke, 7, 327-31

Kannel, W.B. and Gordon, T. (1978) 'Evaluation of Cardiovascular Risk in the Elderly: The Framingham study' Bulletin of the New York Academy of Medicine, 54, 573-91

Karacan, J. and Williams, J. (1983) 'Sleep disorders in the elderly', American Family Physician, 23, 143-52

Kay, D.W.K., Beamish, P. and Roth, M. (1964) 'Old Age Mental Disorders in Newcastle-upon-Tyne', British Journal of Psychiatry, 110, 146-158

Kay, D.W.K., Bergmann, K., Foster, E.M. et al. (1970) 'Mental illness and hospital usage in the elderly', Comprehensive Psychiatry, 11, 26-35

Kellet, J.M. (1984) 'Sleep and the Elderly: A review of sleep disorders in clinical practice', Sleep Topics, 4, 7-8

Kennedy, I. (1983) The Unmasking of Medicine, London, Paladin

Kessel Report (1977) First Report of the Advisory Committee on Alcoholism - Prevention, Department of Health and Social Security, London, HMSO

Kesson, C.M., Gray, J.M.B. and Lawson, D.H. (1976) 'Benzodiozepine drugs in general medical patients', British Medical Journal, i, 680-82

Klotz, U., Avant, G.R., Hoyumpa, A. et al. (1975) 'The effects of age and liver disease on the disposition and elimination of diazepam in adult man', Journal of Clinical Investigation, 55, 347-359

Knox, J.D.E. (1980) 'Prescribing for the elderly in general practice', Journal of the Royal College of General Practitioners, 30, Supplement 1, 1-8

Knox, J.D.E. (1985) 'The limited list and prescribing for the elderly', Geriatric Medicine, April, 1

Kofoed, L.L. (1986) 'OTC drugs: a third of the elderly are at risk', Geriatric Medicine, February, 37-41

Kotin, J., Wilbert, D.E., Verburg, D. and Soldinger

S.M. (1976) 'Thioridazine and sexual dysfunction', American Journal of Psychiatry, 133, 82-85

Kromhout, D., Bosschieter, E. and Conlander, C. (1982) 'Dietary Fibre and 10-Year Mortality from Coronary Heart Disease, Cancer and All Causes: The Zutphen Study', Lancet, ii, 518-523

Laekeman, G.M. (1984) 'Drug information leaflets for patients', Pharmacy International, April, 103-6

Lafaille, R. (1983) 'A New Perspective for Health Care', in Hatch, S. and Kickbusch, I. (eds), Self-help and Health in Europe, Copenhagen, World Health Organisation

Lamy, P.P. (1980a) 'Drug interactions and the elderly - a new perspective', Drug Intelligence and Clinical Pharmacy, 14, 513-15

Lamy, P.P. (1980b) Prescribing for the Elderly, New York, Wright Publishing

Lancet leader (1983) 'Pharmacokinetics in the Elderly', Lancet, i, 568-69

Lancet leader (1984) 'Diet and Hypertension', ii, 671-673

Lancet leader (1985) 'Dietary Potassium and Hypertension', Lancet, i, 308-9

Landahl, S., Lindblad, B. Roupe, S. et al. (1977) 'Digitalis therapy in a 70 year old population', Acta Medica Scandinavia, 202, 437-43

Law, R. and Chalmers, C. (1976) 'Medicines and elderly people: a general practice survey', British Medical Journal, i, 565-68

Learoyd, B.M. (1972) 'Psychotropic drugs and the elderly patient', Medical Journal of Australia, i, 1131-33

Leeson, J. and Gray, J. (1978) Women and Medicine, London, Tavistock Books

Lehr, U. (1983) 'Stereotypes of ageing and age norms', in Birren, J.E., Munnichs, J., Thomae, H. and Marois, M. (eds) Ageing: A Challenge to Science and Society, Oxford University Press, Oxford, pp.101-111

Lewis, J.G. (1984) 'Adverse effects of oral diuretics', Adverse Drug Reaction Bulletin, No. 109, 404-7

Lichtenstein, M. (1985) 'Jogging in Middle Age', Journal of the Royal College of General Practitioners, 35, 341-345

Lindsey, A. (1962) Socialized Medicine in England and Wales, Chapel Hill, The University of North Carolina Press

Linkewich, J.A., Catalano, R.B. and Flock, H.L. (1974) 'The effect of packaging and instruction on outpatient compliance with medication regimes', Drug Intelligence and Clinical Pharmacy, 8, 10-15

Lipton, H. and Lee, P. (forthcoming) Drugs and the Elderly, Stanfor, Standford University Press

Lishman, A.W. (1978) Organic Psychiatry, Oxford, Blackwell Scientific Publications Ltd.

Liverpool Therapeutic Group (1978) 'Use of digitalis in general practice', British Medical Journal, ii, 673-75

Bibliography

Lloyd-Evans, S., Brocklehurst, J.C. and Palmer, M.K. (1978) 'Assessment of drug therapy in chronic brain failure', Gerontology, 24, 304-11

Lorand, A. (1910) Old Age Deferred, Philadelphia, F.A. Davis

Lorig, K. and Fries, J. (1983) The Arthritis Help Book, London, Souvenir Press

Lorig, K., Laurin, J. and Holman, H. (1984) 'Arthritis Self-Management: A Study of the Effectiveness of Patient Education for the Elderly', Gerontologist, 24, 455-57

Macdonald, E.T. and Macdonald, J.B. (1977) 'Nocturnal femoral fracture and continuing wide-spread use of barbiturate hypnotics'. British Medical Journal, ii, 483-85

Macdonald, E.T. and Macdonald, J.B. (1982) Drug treatment in the elderly, Chichester, John Wiley and Sons

Macdonald, E.T., Macdonald, J.B. and Phoenix, M. (1977) 'Improving drug compliance after hospital discharge', British Medical Journal, ii, 618-21

Macfadyen, D. (1985) 'Self-Health Care: International Perspectives', in Glendenning, F. (ed) New Initiatives in Self-Health Care for Older People, Stoke-on-Trent, A Beth Johnson Foundation Publication in association with Keele University Department of Adult Education and the Health Education Council

McGhie, A. and Russell, S.M. (1962) 'The subjective assessment of normal sleep patterns', Journal of Mental Science, 108, 642-54

MacIntyre, S. (1977) 'Old Age as a Social Problem', in Dingwall, R., Health, C., Reid, M. and Stacy, M. Health Care and Health Knowledge, London, Croom Helm

McKinlay, J.B. (ed) (1985) Issues in the Political Economy of Health Care, London, Tavistock

Macleod, C.C., Judge, T.G. and Caird, F.I. (1975) 'Nutrition of Elderly at Home: Intake of Minerals', Age and Ageing, 4, 49-57

MacMahon, S.W., Macdonald, G.J., Bernstein, L. et al. (1985) 'Comparison of weight reduction with metoprolol in treatment of hypertension in young overweight patients', Lancet, ii, 1233-36

McManners, J. (1985) Death and the Enlightenment, Oxford, Oxford University Press

Manek, S., Rutherford, J., Jackson, S.H.D. and Turner, P. (1984) 'Persistence of divergent views of hospital staff in detecting and managing hypertension', British Medical Journal, 289, 1433-34

Mann, A.H., Jenkins, R., Cross, P.S. and Gurland, B.J. (1984) 'A comparison of the prescriptions received by the elderly in long-term care in New York and London', Psychological Medicine, 14, 891-97

Marks, J. (1984) 'How to take care with benzodiazepines',

168

Rational Prescriber, No 4, 1-3

Martinsen, E., Medhus, A., and Sandvik, L. (1985) 'Effects of aerobic exercise on depression: a controlled study', British Medical Journal, 291, 109

Martys, C.R. (1979) 'Adverse reactions to drugs in general practice', British Medical Journal, ii, 1194-97

Means, R. and Smith, R. (1985) The Development of Welfare Services for Elderly People, London, Croom Helm

Medawar, C. (1984) The wrong kind of medicine?, London, Consumers' Association and Hodder and Stoughton

Medical Research Council (1977) 'Working Party on Mild to Moderate Hypertension: Randomised controlled trial of treatment for mild hypertension: design and potential', British Medical Journal, ii, 1437-40

Medical Research Council (1985) 'MRC Trial treatment of mild hypertension: principal results', British Medical Journal, 291, 97-104

Melville, A. and Johnson, C. (1982) 'Cured to death: The effect of prescription drugs', London, New English Library

Michel, K. and Kolakowska, T. (1981) 'A Survey of Prescribing Psychotropic Drugs in Two Psychiatric Hospitals', British Journal of Psychiatry, 138, 217-21

Midlands Bank (1985) 'Prospects for the Pharmaceutical Industry', Midlands Bank Review, Summer, 7-16

Millson, D., Bolland, C., Murphy, P. and Davison, W. (1984) 'Accumulation of midazolam in patients receiving mechanical ventilation' (letter), British Medical Journal, 289, 1308-1309

MIND (1979) Mental Health of Elderly People, London, Mind

Ministry of Health (1962) A Hospital Plan for England and Wales, Cmnd 1604, London, HMSO

Mitchinson, M.J. (1980) 'The hypotensive stroke', Lancet, i, 244-48

Morgan, H.G. (1984) 'Do minor affective disorders need medication?', British Medical Journal, 289, 783

Morgan, K. (1982) 'Effect of Low dose nitrazepam on performance in the elderly', Lancet, i, 516

Morgan, K. and Gilleard, C.J. (1981) 'Patterns of hypnotic prescribing and usage in residential homes for the elderly', Neuropharmacology Journal, 20, 1355-56

Morris, J.N., Marr, J.W., Clayton, D.G. (1977) 'Diet and Heart: a postcript', British Medical Journal, ii, 1307-14

Morton, W. (1956) 'Hospital Care of the Elderly', in Hobson, W. (ed) Introduction to Modern Geriatrics, London, Butterworth

Moules, G. (1984) 'Tune in to better reception', World Medicine, September, 36

Murphy, E. (1983) 'The prognosis of depression in old age', British Journal of Psychiatry, 142, 111-19

Myers, E.D. and Calvert, E.J. (1978) 'Knowledge of side

effects and perseverence with medication', British Journal of Psychiatry, 132, 526-27

National Union of Public Employees (1985) (Wales Division), Dignity or Despair, NUPE

Neis, A., Robinson, D.S., Friedman, M.J. et al. (1977) 'Relationship between age and tricyclic antidepressant plasma levels', American Journal of Psychiatry, 134, 790-93

Neumann, H.H. (1979) 'Sleeping pills' (letter), New England Journal of Medicine, 301, 214

Nuki, G. (1983) 'Non-Steroidal analgesic and anti-inflammatory agents', British Medical Journal, 287, 39-43

Oakley, A. (1984) The Captive Womb, Oxford, Basil Blackwell

O'Brien, E., Fitzgerald, D. and O'Malley, K. (1985) 'Blood pressure measurements, current practice and future trends', British Medical Journal, 290, 729-33

Office of Health Economics (OHE) (1977) Sources of Information for Prescribing Doctors in Britain, London, OHE

Office of Health Economics (OHE) (1980) A Question of Balance: the benefits and risks of pharmaceutical innovation, London, OHE

Office of Health Economics (OHE) (1983) Keep on taking the tablets? A review of the problem of patient non-compliance, Briefing No 21, London, OHE

OPCS (1984) General Household Survey 1982, London, HMSO

OPCS (1985) 'Cigarette Smoking 1972 to 1984', London, OPCS Monitor, Reference GHS 85/2

O'Malley, K. (1985) 'New light on management of hypertension', Geriatric Medicine, 15, 13-17

O'Malley, K., Crooks, J., Duke, E. and Stevenson, I.H. (1971) 'Effect of age and sex on human drug metabolism', British Medical Journal, iii, 607-9

O'Malley, K. and O'Brien, E. (1980) 'Management of hypertension in the elderly', New England Journal of Medicine, 302, 1397-1401

Opren Action Committee (1985) 'Briefing on Benoxaprofen (Opren)', Mimeo

Orme, E. (1955) My Fight Against Osteoarthritis, London, Faber and Faber

Oswald, I. (1984a) 'Symptoms that depress the doctor: Insomnia', British Journal of Hospital Medicine, 31, 219-24

Oswald, I. (1984b) 'Limiting prescribable NHS drugs', British Medical Journal, 289, 1536

Oswald, I. and Adam, K. (1980) 'Benzodiazepines cause small loss of body weight', British Medical Journal, 281, 1039-40

Oswald, I. and Priest, R. (1965) 'Five weeks to escape the sleeping pill habit', British Medical Journal, ii, 1093-95

Overstall, P.W. (1982) 'Treatment of sleep disturbances in the elderly', in Wheatley, D. (ed) Psychopharmacology of Old Age, Oxford University Press, pp.171-176

Parish, P. (1971) 'The prescribing of psychotropic drugs in general practice', Journal of the Royal College of General Practitioners, 21, supplement 4: 1-77

Parish, P., Dogett, M.A. and Colleypriest, P. (1983) The elderly and their use of medicines, Kings Fund project paper No 40, London, Kings Fund

Parish, P. and Weedle, P. (1984) 'Pharmacists' responsibility for the care of the elderly', British Journal of Pharmaceutical Practice, November, 346

Parkin, D.M., Henney, C.R., Quirk, J. and Crooks, J. (1976) 'Deviation from prescribed treatment after discharge from hospital', British Medical Journal, ii, 686-88

Parkin, D.M., Kellett, R.J., Maclean, D.W. et al. (1979) 'The management of hypertension, a study of records in general practice', Journal of the Royal College of General Practitioners, 29, 590-94

Parr, J. (1951) How I Cured my Duodenal Ulcer, London, Michael Joseph

Parrott, A.C. and Kentridge, R. (1982) 'Personal constructs of anxiety under the 1,5 - benzodiazepine clobazam related to trait-anxiety levels of the personality', Psychopharmacology, 78, 353-57

Paton, A. (1984) 'Doctors and the Drug Makers', THS Health Summary, 1, 8

Perri, S. and Templer, D. (1985) 'The Effects of an Aerobic Exercise Program on Psychological Variables in Older Adults', International Journal of Aging and Human Development, 20, 167-172

Petrie, J.C., Robb, O.J., Webster, J. et al. (1985) 'Computer assisted shared care in hypertension', British Medical Journal, 290, 1960-62

Peturrson, H. and Lader, M.H. (1981) 'Benzodiazepine dependence', British Journal of Addiction, 76, 133-45

Pharmaceutical Society (1986) The Administration and Control of Medicines in Residential Homes, London, Pharmaceutical Society

Phillipson, C. (1981) 'Pre-Retirement Education: The British amd American Experience', Ageing and Society, 1, 393-414

Phillipson, C. (1982) Capitalism and the Construction of Old Age, London, Macmillan Books

Phillipson, C. (1983) Drugs and the Elderly: A Critical Perspective on the Opren Case, Critical Social Policy, 3, 109-116

Phillipson C. and Strang, P. (1983) The Impact of Pre-Retirement Education: a longitudinal evaluation, Stoke-on-Trent, Department of Adult Education, University of Keele

Phillipson, C. and Strang, P. (1984) Health Education and Older People: The Role of Paid Carers, Stoke-on-Trent, Health Education Council in association with Department of Adult and Continuing Education, University of Keele

Phillipson, C. and Strang, P. (1986) Training and Education for an Ageing Society: Perspectives for the Health and Social Services, Stoke-on-Trent, Health Education Council in association with the Department of Adult and Continuing Education, University of Keele

Phillipson, C. and Walker, A. (1986) Ageing and Social Policy: A Critical Assessment, Aldershot, Gower Press

Pickup, A.J., Mee, L.G. and Hedley, A.J. (1983) 'The general practitioner and continuing education', Journal of the Royal College of General Practitioners, 33, 486-490

Plant, J. (1977) 'Educating the Elderly in Safe Medication Use', Journal of the American Hospital Association, 51, 97-101

Political and Economic Planning (PEP) (1948) Population Policy in Great Britain, London, PEP

Porter, R. (1984) 'Do We Really Need Doctors', New Society, 69, 87-89

Porter, R. (1985) 'The Patient's View: Doing Medical History from Below', Theory and Society, 14, 167-174

Power, K.G., Jerrom, D.W.A., Simpson, R.J. and Mitchell, M. (1985) 'Controlled study of withdrawal symptoms and rebound anxiety after six week course of diazepam for generalised anxiety', British Medical Journal, 290, 1246-48

Prescott, L. (1979) 'Factors predisposing of adverse drug reactions', Adverse Drug Reaction Bulletin, No 78, 280-83

Prescott, L. and Highley, M.S. (1985) 'Drugs prescribed for self poisoners', British Medical Journal, 290, 1633-36

Puska, P. et al. (1983) 'Controlled, Randomised Trial of the Effect of Dietary Fat in Blood Pressure', Lancet, i, 1-5

Ramsay, L.E. (1984) 'Diuretics and antihypertensive drugs', Prescribers Journal, 24, 60-65

Ramus, C. (1926) Outwitting Middle Age, New York, Century

Ratna, L. (1981) 'Addiction to temazepam', British Medical Journal, 282, 1837-38

Rawlins, M. (1984) 'Doctors and the Drug Makers', The Lancet, ii, 276-278

Rice, D. and Arie, T. (1981) 'Drugs for anxiety and depression in the elderly', MIMS Magazine, 15 June, 51-57

Richards, P. (1979) 'Drug induced metabolic disease', British Medical Journal, i, 1128-29

Riessman, F., Moody, H.R. and Worthy, E.H. (1984) 'Self-Help and the Elderly', Social Policy, 14, 19-26

Riska, E. and Klaukka, T. (1984) 'Use of psychotropic drugs in Finland', Social Science and Medicine, 19, 983-989

Roberts, H. (1985) The Patient Patients: Women and Their Doctors, London, Pandora Press

Rogers, H.J., Spector, R.G. and Trounce, J.R. (1981) A Textbook of Clinical Pharmacology, London, Hodder and Stoughton

Roland, M.O., Zander, L.I., Evans, M. et al. (1985) 'Evaluation of a computer-assisted repeat prescribing programme in general practice', British Medical Journal, 291, 956-958

Rouse, I.L. and Beilin, L.J. (1984) 'Vegetarian diet and blood pressure', Journal of Hypertension, 2, 231-240

Rouse, I.L., Beilin, L.J., Armstrong, B.K. and Vandongen, R. (1983) 'Blood pressure lowering effect of a vegetarian diet: controlled trial in normotensive subjects', Lancet, i, 5-10

Rowlings, C. (1981) Social Work with Elderly People, London, Allen and Unwin

Royal College of Physicians (1981) 'Organic Mental Impairment in the Elderly', Journal of the Royal College of Physicians of London, 15, 1-29

Royal College of Physicians (1983) Report of Working Party on Obesity, Journal of the Royal College of Physicians of London, 17, no.1

Royal College of Physicians (1984) 'Medication for the Elderly', Journal of the Royal College of Physicians of London, 18, 7-17

Royal Commission on Population (1949) Report on Population, Cmnd 7659, London, HMSO

Rudd, T.N. (1972) 'Prescribing methods and the iatrogenic situation in old age', Gerontologica Clinica, 14, 123-28

Sadgrove, J. (1985) 'Women and Smoking', New Statesman, 109, 9-11

Sainsbury Report (1967) Report of the Committee of Enquiry into the Relationship of the Pharmaceutical Industry with the National Health Service, Cmnd. 3410, London, HMSO

Savo, C. (1984) Self-Care and Self-Help Programmes for Older Adults in the United States, Stoke-on-Trent, Health Education Council in association with the Department of Adult and Continuing Education, University of Keele

Sharpe, D. and Kay, M. (1977) 'Worrying trends in prescribing', Modern Geriatrics, 7, 32-36

Shaw, S.M. and Opit, L.J. (1976) 'Need for supervision in the elderly receiving long term prescribed medicines', British Medical Journal, i, 505-7

Shephard, R.J. (1978) Physical Activity and Ageing, London, Croom Helm

Shepherd, M., Cooper, B., Brown, A.C. and Kalton, C. (1966) Psychiatric illness in general practice, Oxford, Oxford University Press

Shulman, J. (1982) 'Pills and Profits: dealing with the drug companies', Medicine in Society, 8, (3), 18-22

Shulman, J. (1983a) 'The Opren Affair - tragedy or scandal?', Medicine in Society, 9, (1), 26-31

Shulman, J. (1983b) 'The Safety of Medicines', Medicine in Society, 9, (3), 7-10

Shulman, J. (1983c) Prevention of adverse drug reactions. Update, 15 October, 1127-1126

Shulman, S., and Shulman, J.I. (1980) 'Operating a two-card medication record system in general practice pharmacy', Practitioner, 224, 989-92

Skegg, D.C.G., Doll, R. and Perry, J. (1977) 'Use of medicines in general practice', British Medical Journal, i, 1561-63

Skegg, D.C.G., Richards, S.M. and Doll, R. (1979) 'Minor tranquillisers and road accidents', British Medical Journal, i, 917-19

Skoll, S.L., August, R.J. Johnson, G.E. et al. (1979) 'Drug Prescribing for the Elderly in Saskatchewan druing 1976', Canadian Medical Association Journal, 121, 1074-81

Sloan, P.J.M. (1984) 'Survey of patient information booklets', British Medical Journal, 288, 915-19

Smith, A.J. (1972) 'Self poisoning with drugs: a worsening situation', British Medical Journal, ii, 157-59

Smith, R. (1985) 'Exercise and Osteoporosis', British Medical Journal, 290, 1163-1164

Smith, S. and Swash, M. (1982) 'Effect of Physostigine on responses in memory tests in patients with Alzheimers Disease', Aging, 19, in Corkin, S., Davis, K.L., Growden, J.H. and Wurlan, R.J. (eds), New York, Raven Press, pp.405-412

Snaith, P. (1983) 'Panic disorders', British Medical Journal, 286, 1376-77

Somerville, K., Faulkner, G. and Langman, M. (1986) 'Non Steroidal Anti-inflammatory Drugs and Bleeding Peptic Ulcer', Lancet, i, 462-464

Spiers, C.J., Griffin, J.P., Weber, J.C.P. et al. (1984) 'Demography of the UK adverse reactions register of spontaneous reports', Health Trends, No. 3, 16, 49-52

Sprakling, M.E., Mitchell, J.R.A., Short, A.H. and Watt, G. (1981) 'Blood pressure reduction in the elderly: A randomised controlled trial of methyldopa', British Medical Journal, 283, 1151-53

Stahl, M.S. and Potts, M.K. (1985) 'Social Support and Chronic Diseases: A Propositional Inventory', in Peterson, W. and Quandango, J. Social Bonds in Later Life, London, Sage Publications, pp.305-324

Stearns, P. (1977) Old Age in European Society: The Case of France, London, Croom Helm

Stephen, P.J. and Williamson, J. (1984) 'Drug induced Parkinsonism in the elderly', Lancet, ii, 1082-3

Stieglitz, E. (1949) The Second Forty Years, London, Staples

Press

Stimson, G. (1974) 'Obeying Doctor's Orders: A View from the Other Side', Social Science and Medicine, 8, 97-104

Stimson, G. (1976) 'The use of references in drug advertisements: Prescribing in general practice', Journal of the Royal College of General Practitioners, Supplement No. 1, 26, 76-80

Subhan, Z. (1983) 'The effect of benzodiazepines on short term memory capacity', in Benzodiazepines Sleep and Day Time Performance, Oxford, The Medicine Publishing Foundation Symposium Series 10, pp.29-42

Subhan, Z. (1984) 'Benzodiazepines and memory', Psychiatry in Practice, 3, 15-19

Swales, J.D. (1985) 'Salt and blood pressure', Update, March 1, 407-415

Swash, M. (1983) 'Alzheimer's disease', The Physcian 1, 341-43

Swift, C.G. (1982) 'Hypnotic drugs' in Isaacs, B. (ed) Recent Advances in Geriatric Medicine, Vol 2, Edinburgh, Churchill Livingstone, pp.123-146

Swift, C.G. et al. (1980) 'Single dose effects of oral diazepam in the elderly', in Turner, P. and Padgham, C. (Abstracts from) World Conference on Clinical Pharmacology and Therapeutics, London, Macmillan

Szabadi, E. (1984) 'Neuroleptic malignant syndrome', British Medical Journal, 288, 1399-1400

Taylor, D. (1983) 'Medicine for the elderly', Journal of the Market Research Society, 25, 263-74

Taylor, P. (1984) The Smoke Ring: Tobacco, Money and Multinational Politics, London, Sphere Books

Thompson, K. (1986) 'The case for developmental gerontology - Thompson's Octad', Journal of the Royal College of General Practitioners, 36, 29-32

Thornton, E.W. (1985) Exercise and Ageing: An Unproven Relationship, Liverpool, Liverpool University Press

Toghill, P.J., Smith, P.G., Beuton, P. et al. (1974) 'Methyldopa liver damage', British Medical Journal, iii, 545-548

Tomlinson, B.E., Blessed, G. and Roth, M. (1970) 'Observations on the brains of demented old people', Journal of the Neurological Sciences, 11, 205-242

Townsend, P. (1964) The Last Refuge: A Survey of Residential Institutions and Homes for the Aged in England and Wales, London, Routledge and Kegan Paul

Townsend, P. (1981) 'The Structured Dependency of the Elderly: Creation of Social Policy in the Twentieth Century', Ageing and Society, 1, 5-29

Townsend, P. and Davidson, N. (eds) (1982) Inequalities in Health, London, Pelican Books

Truswell, A.S. (1985a) 'Diet and Hypertension', British Medical Journal, 291, 125-127

Truswell, A.S. (1985b) 'Reducing the Risk of Coronary Heart Disease', British Medical Journal, 291, 34-37

Tuft, N. (1982) 'Polypharmacy rules but pill pushing amongst pensioners isn't OK', New Age, Issue No.19, 14-16

Tyrer, P. (1978) 'Drug treatment of psychiatric patients in general practice', British Medical Journal, ii, 1008-10

Tyrer, P. (1984a) 'Classification of anxiety', British Journal of Psychiatry, 144, 78-83

Tyrer, P. (1984b) 'Benzodiazepines on trial', British Medical Journal, 288, 1101-2

Tyrer, P., Owen, R. and Dawling, S. (1983) 'Gradual withdrawal of diazepam after long term therapy', Lancet, i, 1402-6

Varnam, M.A. (1981) 'Psychotropic prescribing. What am I doing?', Journal of the Royal College of General Practitioners, 31, 480-83

Velasquez, M.J. and Hoffman, R. (1985) 'Overweight and Obesity in Hypertension', Quarterly Journal of Medicine, New series, 54, 205-212

Vestel, R.E. (1978) 'Drug Use in the Elderly: A Review of Problems and Special Considerations', Drugs, 16, 358-382

Vetter, N.J., Jones, D.A. and Victor, C.R. (1985) 'Use of medications on the restricted list by the elderly', British Medical Journal, 290, 1712-3

Wade, B. and Finlayson, J. (1983) 'Drugs and the elderly', Nursing Mirror, May 4, 17-21

Wade, B.E., Sawyer, L. and Bell, J. (1983) Dependency with dignity, Occasional Papers on Social Administration No. 68, Bedford Square Press, London

Walker, C. and Cannon, G. (1985) The Food Scandal, London, Century Publishing

Walker, I. (1983) 'Institutional Care: The Creation of a Learning Environment', in Johnstone, S. and Phillipson, C. (eds) Older Learners: The Challenge to Adult Education, London, Bedford Square Press

Walker, A. (1985) The Care Gap: How can local authorities meet the needs of the elderly, London, Local Government Information Unit

Walt, R., Katschinski, B., Locan, R. et al. (1986) 'Rising Frequency of Ulcer Perforation in Elderly People in the United Kingdom', The Lancet, i, 489-493

Wandless, I. and Davie, J.W.L. (1977) 'Can drug compliance in the elderly be improved?', British Medical Journal, i, 359-61

de Wardener, H.E. (1984) 'Salt and Hypertension', Lancet, ii, 688

Watson, C. (1913) The Book of Diet, London, Thomas Nelson

Webb, A.L. and Hobdell, M. (1980) 'Co-ordination and Teamwork in the Health and Personal Social Services', in Lonsdale, S., Webb, A.L. and Briggs, J.L. (eds), Teamwork in the Personal Social Services and Health

Care, London, Croom Helm

Weedle, P. and Parish, P. (1984 and 1985) 'Pharmaceutical Care of the Elderly', British Journal of Pharmaceutical Practice, November and subsequent issues to June

Whiting, B., Wandless, I., Sumner, D.J. and Goldberg, A. (1978) 'A computer assisted review of digoxin therapy in the elderly', British Heart Journal, 40, 8-13

Wilkin, D. (1983) 'General Practitioners and the Elderly', Mimeo, Paper to the British Society of Gerontology Annual Conference, University of Liverpool

Williams, B.O. (1985) 'Use and misuse of diuretics in the elderly', Prescribers Journal, 25, 51-56

Williams, P. (1980) 'Recent trends in the prescribing of psychotropic drugs', Health Trends, 12, 6-7

Williams, P. (1983a) 'Factors influencing the duration of treatment with psychotropic drugs in general practice: survival analysis approach', Psychological Medicine, 13, 623-33

Williams, P. (1983b) 'Patterns of psychotropic drug use', Social Science and Medicine, 17, 845-51

Williams, P.T., Wood, P.D., Haskell, W.L. and Vranizen, K. (1982) 'The effects of running mileage and duration on plasma lipoprotein levels', Journal of American Medicine, 247, 2674-2679

Williamson, J. (1978) 'Prescribing problems in the elderly', Practitioner, 220, 749-55

Williamson, J. (1984) 'Drug induced Parkinsons Disease', British Medical Journal, 288, 1457

Williamson, J. and Chopin, J.M. (1980) 'Adverse reactions to prescribed drugs in the elderly: a multi-centre investigation', Age and Ageing, 9, 73-80

Williamson, J., Stokoe, I.H., Gray, S. et al. (1964) 'Old people at home: their unreported needs', Lancet, i, 1117-20

Williamson, J.W., Aaronovitch, S., Simonson, L. et al. (1975) 'Health accounting, an outcome based system of quality assurance: Illustrative application to hypertension', Bulletin of the New York Academy of Medicine, 51, 727-38

Wilson, C.W., Banks, J.A., Mapes, R. and Korte, S. (1963) 'Influence of Different Sources of Therapeutic Information on Prescribing by General Practitioners', British Medical Journal, ii, 599-604

Wollner, L., McCarthy, S.T., Soper, N.D.W. and Macy, D.J. (1979) 'Failure of cerebral autoregulation as a cause of brain dysfunction in the elderly', British Medical Journal, i, 1117-18

Women's National Commission (1984) Women and the Health Service, London, The Cabinet Office

World Health Organisation (1981) The Control of Drugs for the Elderly, WHO Report, Copenhagen, WHO

Bibliography

World Health Organisation (1985) Drugs for the Elderly,
(available from HMSO Publications, London)
Wright, J.M., McLeod, P.J. and McCullogh, W. (1976)
'Antihypertensive efficacy of a single bedtime dose of
methyldopa', Clinical Pharmacology and Therapeutics, 20,
733-37
Young, A. (1984) 'Exercise against disease, disuse and
disability', Update, October, 531-538
Zola, I. (1978) 'Medicine as an institution of social control', in
Ehrenreich, J. (ed) The Cultural Crisis of Modern
Medicine, New York, Monthly Review Press

INDEX

For Product Safety Concerns and Information please contact our EU
representative GPSR@taylorandfrancis.com
Taylor & Francis Verlag GmbH, Kaufingerstraße 24, 80331 München, Germany